THE SKINCARE BIBLE

THE SKINCARE BIBLE
Your No-Nonsense Guide to Great Skin

DR ANJALI MAHTO

PENGUIN LIFE

AN IMPRINT OF

PENGUIN BOOKS

PENGUIN LIFE

UK | USA | Canada | Ireland | Australia
India | New Zealand | South Africa

Penguin Life is part of the Penguin Random House group of companies
whose addresses can be found at global.penguinrandomhouse.com.

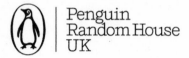

First published 2018

009

Set in 12.5/16 pt Dante MT Std
Typeset by Jouve (UK), Milton Keynes
Printed and bound in Great Britain by Clays Ltd, Elcograf S.p.A.

A CIP catalogue record for this book is available from the British Library

ISBN: 978–0–241–30910–0

www.greenpenguin.co.uk

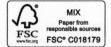

MIX
Paper from
responsible sources
FSC
www.fsc.org   FSC® C018179

Penguin Random House is committed to a
sustainable future for our business, our readers
and our planet. This book is made from Forest
Stewardship Council® certified paper.

For my parents, Baidya Nath and Kamla Mahto

CONTENTS

INTRODUCTION

The UK beauty market is worth £17 billion, a figure that is likely to rise in the coming years and decades due to the increasing amount we are willing to spend on products and our changing lifestyles. The desire to have flawless, youthful skin is not new and has been documented since the times of Ancient Egypt, when unguent, a soothing ointment, was popularly used to hydrate the skin and kohl to decorate the eyes.

In some ways, it is surprising how little has changed over the centuries in terms of our ideals of beauty. The holy grail of perfect skin still remains very much on our modern-day radar. Rightly or wrongly, blemish-free skin is still seen as an outward marker for good health and well-being.

The media bombards us from an early age with societal ideals of beauty. The portrayal of seemingly unachievable perfection still pervades glossy magazines and newspapers, accentuated further by heavily filtered and edited social media feeds. Who isn't guilty of scrolling through Instagram only to be assailed by image after image of picture-perfect celebrities with their picture-perfect skin? Whilst we should know better, more often than not it is easy to be taken in by what we see and read; those celebrities are people too, and also suffer from the same skin afflictions that blight the rest of us mere mortals.

One thing that has really struck me over the years is how much my attitude to what I read about skincare has changed. As a teenager in the early 90s, suffering dreadful acne, I hungrily read every magazine I could get my hands on that would offer me a 'cure'. Let me get this straight from the outset: apple cider vinegar, home-made sugar scrubs, toothpaste, TCP and peel-off masks didn't work (and this is just the tip of the iceberg!). The acne, of course, improved after seeing a dermatologist – not due to any of the hundreds of skincare products I had wasted my money on. You would think I would have learned my lesson . . . but no. I still turned to the same magazines when it came to treating my acne scars. Unsurprisingly, lavender oil was not an adequate treatment for the ice pick scarring on my cheeks.

Over the years, I finished my dermatology training and developed an interest in beauty and skincare in addition to my focus on medical skin problems. I was still reading the same types of magazines, but was now able to critically appraise both the treatments that were being promoted and the doctors or experts that were being quoted. I realized that beauty magazines have close relationships with PR companies. PR companies work for beauty and skincare producers. These beauty and skincare producers, in turn, pay PR companies vast sums of money to promote themselves and their products. So, a lot of what we read in the magazines is indirectly sponsored, and it's difficult for us to tell the advertising apart from the sound medical advice.

The bottom line is this: often, the 'experts' are not really the experts.

This creates an absolute minefield for anyone that just wants sound, unbiased skincare advice backed by science. The latest new beauty trend from Korea – is it a fad or is there genuinely something useful in the concept? Combine the glossy magazines and style sections of the newspapers and throw in the fact that anyone can blog about anything. Everyone has an opinion on skincare and what they feel works. How can anyone spot the proven treatments from the next money-spinning product?

This book provides quality advice on skin and skincare. It is inspired by exactly the kinds of questions I get asked on a daily basis in my outpatient clinic by people just like you and me. The advice provides clarity in the face of the multitude of conflicting messages that bombard us from all sides. We should be empowered to question what we read and learn to reject the information provided to us that is bereft of a sound scientific basis.

More than that, I hope this book will provide a lifeline to those that have been struggling with their skin for years or simply have not had the confidence to seek help. Skin issues are recognized causes of low self-esteem, anxiety, depression and social isolation. This can trigger a vicious cycle in which the psychological issues that develop only further exacerbate the skin problem. Arming you with an accurate source of information and the knowledge of when to seek medical advice may help in part to break this cycle down.

The monolith of misinformation about this beautiful, complex organ needs to be shattered. Good skin can be achieved by all of us – not just the lucky few with good genes, plenty of time or big money on their hands. Quality skincare does not have to be complicated or expensive and it is never too late to start or mix up your skincare routine. The time is now to make your skin your priority.

1

A CRASH COURSE IN SKIN

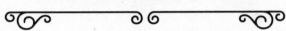

It's impossible to understand skincare without first understanding a bit about the skin and how it works. In this chapter, I'm going to try to distil the basics from what is quite elaborate science to give you everything you need to know.

Human skin is a complex biological organ straddling the junction between beauty, health and disease. Rightly or wrongly, good skin, particularly of the face, has long been considered a marker of attractiveness. It is closely linked not just to the visual aesthetic, but also to self-esteem, confidence and how we view ourselves.

Skin, however, is more than just skin-deep. Our skin has a number of important physiological roles in maintaining health: it provides a physical and biochemical barrier to the outside world, simultaneously protecting us from ultraviolet (UV) light from the sun, preventing water loss and blocking the entry of unwanted microbes and chemicals. Cells of the immune system are ubiquitous in the skin, preventing infection. Body temperature is regulated by blood vessels in the skin. Skin is a vital sensory organ and site of vitamin D production. We can become so obsessed with making our skin look good that we forget to thank it for all the amazing things it does for us every day.

SKIN STRUCTURE

To understand exactly how beauty products work, why common skin problems occur and what happens to our skin as it ages, it is important to have a basic understanding of normal skin structure and its constituent components.

The skin has two main parts: the upper epidermis and the lower dermis. These together sit on top of a layer of fat and connective tissue that gives the skin its support.

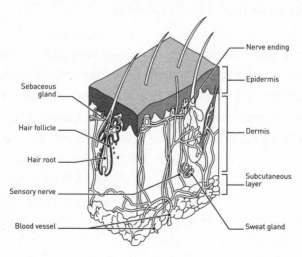

The outermost layer of the skin – the upper part of the epidermis – is known as the stratum corneum. This is made up of dead skin cells that are integral to the skin's function as a barrier. Skin cells turn over approximately every twenty-eight days, with cells from the upper layers being continually shed and replaced by cells from deeper layers.

The epidermis

The epidermis is the outermost part of the skin, the bit that gets up close and personal with the outside world. To do its job successfully as the first line of defence, it has four main cell types, each with its own important role to play.

a) Keratinocytes

The main cell in the epidermis, keratinocytes produce the protein keratin, which provides the skin with physical protection and waterproofing. You may already be familiar with keratin as it's also the main component of hair and nails, and can also be an ingredient in some personal-care products.

b)   Melanocytes

These cells produce the pigment melanin, which gives our skin its colour and protects us against UV light from the sun.

c)   Langerhans cells

Langerhans cells are part of the immune system and are ready to seek and destroy any microbes that may invade the skin.

d)   Merkel cells

These sensory cells are found deep in the epidermis, and provide us with the sensation of touch.

The dermis

The dermis sits below the epidermis. It is often divided into two layers: the upper 'papillary' dermis and the lower 'reticular' dermis. The papillary dermis is rich in nerve endings whilst the reticular dermis provides the skin with its structural support and elasticity, and is rich in collagen, elastin and hyaluronic acid. The beauty industry and anti-ageing market has taken much interest in these molecules, and as the terms are often thrown about in writing and talk on skincare, they definitely warrant a closer look.

a)   Collagen

Collagen is one of the most abundant proteins in the body. It forms a scaffold that gives strength, rigidity and support to the skin. There are at least sixteen different types of collagen in the skin, although 80 to 90 per cent of human collagen is of types 1, 2 and 3. Gram for gram, collagen is stronger than steel.

b)   Elastin

Elastin is another connective tissue protein found in skin. As its name suggests, elastin gives skin its elasticity; indeed, its properties are often compared to those of elastic bands: it allows skin to resume its original shape after being stretched, pinched or poked.

c)   Hyaluronic acid

Hyaluronic acid belongs to a group of compounds known as glycosaminoglycans, and also forms part of the skin's framework. It is essentially a very large sugar molecule with a gel-like consistency. Hyaluronic acid has a unique capacity to bind over 1,000 times its own weight in water. Its purpose in skin is to keep it soft, plump and hydrated. Hyaluronic acid is a popular constituent in skincare due to its moisturizing properties; it can also be injected into, or under, the skin in the form of dermal fillers.

SKIN AGEING

The process of getting older outwardly can be seen in the skin before any other organ of the body. Changes are visible to us and to those around us and growing old cannot be hidden, unlike many other medical issues. We are living longer than ever before and, for some people, the natural changes associated with skin ageing can be seen as undesirable or even unhealthy. The anti-ageing market continues to grow in lockstep with this, often in response to (but also frequently driving) exactly these kinds of concerns.

The science behind skin ageing

As skin ages, there is a reduction in both the number and size of skin cells. It functions less effectively as a protective barrier, temperature regulation is less efficient and there is a decline in the production of sweat, sebum (oil) and vitamin D. The skin itself becomes increasingly thin over time due to a steady reduction in collagen, elastin and hyaluronic acid (it is commonly quoted that collagen production in the skin falls by 1 per cent each year after the age of twenty). Cells turn over less quickly and wound healing is relatively impaired.

To the external observer, these changes become apparent as dry skin, fine lines, deep furrows and wrinkles. Skin starts to sag as it loses its support and textural changes appear. Broken blood vessels, thread veins and uneven skin pigmentation become more prominent. Frighteningly, some of these changes can set in as early as your late twenties or early thirties. Aesthetics aside, ageing also affects the skin's immune response and certain skin cancers become more common as we get older.

WHAT CAUSES SKIN AGEING?

Skin ageing occurs for a variety of reasons; some of these are under our control (extrinsic factors) whilst others are not (intrinsic factors). Let's look at these in more detail.

Intrinsic ageing

Intrinsic, or 'chronological', skin ageing is inevitable and, with our current understanding, cannot be prevented in practice; it happens to all of us and is largely genetically determined. If your parents aged well, the chances are good that you will also. We have learned much about the mechanisms of ageing in recent years and a number of underlying causes have been hypothesized. These include:

a)   Telomere shortening

Our DNA is tightly packaged into thread-like structures called chromosomes. Telomeres are specialized regions found at the ends of chromosomes and are analogous to the plastic tips found at the ends of shoelaces. Telomeres prevent the ends of the chromosomes fraying or sticking to one another. Each time a cell divides, its telomeres get shorter, and when they get too short, the cell is no longer able to divide; it consequently becomes inactive or dies. This process of telomere shortening has been linked to skin ageing as well as certain human diseases. Although there is a lot of ongoing research in this area, we don't yet understand telomeres well enough to develop a safe cure for telomere shortening.

b) Mitochondrial damage

Mitochondria are the tiny 'powerhouses' inside human cells, converting oxygen and nutrients into the chemical energy that powers them. Energy production generates free radicals, harmful molecules which have the ability to damage the cell itself over time and if allowed to accumulate. The processes by which mitochondria generate energy, therefore, also have the ability to damage it, rendering cells past their 'sell-by' date.

c) Hormonal changes

Hormonal changes, particularly in women, are also thought to contribute to intrinsic skin ageing. Women are more vulnerable to hormonally induced ageing than men due to the more complex hormonal patterns that occur not just over the course of their monthly cycles, but also during their lifetime as a whole. After the menopause, levels of the hormone oestrogen decline. This has been linked to a loss of skin elasticity, reduced hydration and reduced water-binding capacity. Skin changes are noticeably significant after the menopause.

Extrinsic ageing

Now, extrinsic factors are the ones we have the ability to control or change. Extrinsic ageing occurs against the background of intrinsic ageing. And whilst I love basking in the summer heat, UVA and UVB rays in sunlight are the biggest culprits implicated in the skin's extrinsic ageing process. Sunlight also contains other wavelengths of light, including infrared-A and high-energy visible light, and recent data suggests that these may also have a lesser role to play. So, if you want to keep your youthful good looks, sun protection is an absolute must.

To put all this into perspective, the effects of sunlight are thought to contribute a whopping 80 to 90 per cent of the visible signs associated with ageing. These include wrinkles, pigmentation, sunspots and reduced skin elasticity. Compare the skin on your buttocks or upper inner forearms to the skin on your face or hands. The latter are subject to chronic sun exposure and are much more likely than the former two sites to show, with age, features such as wrinkles or pigmentation. Scientific research on sets of identical twins confirms that the twin with more sun exposure shows features of skin ageing much earlier. As they are genetically identical, we can be confident that the difference was due to the environmental factor: the sun exposure.

So let's look at ultraviolet light in a bit more detail, seeing as it's the cause of many of our ageing woes. UVA is the predominant ray and the ratio of UVA to UVB rays is on average 20:1. This may come as a surprise, but UVA has the ability to penetrate clouds and window glass, causing damage to the skin. This is something to think about if you spend a lot of time driving or near windows.

The proportion of UVA reaching the earth's surface is relatively constant throughout the year, but due to environmental factors such as cloud cover, the proportion of UVB reaching the earth's surface peaks in the summer months. In the UK, due to our latitude, there is very little UVB in the winter months.

The different types of UV light interact with our skin at different depths. UVB rays, with a shorter wavelength than UVA, mostly penetrate the upper skin layers or epidermis; it is UVB that primarily causes skin reddening and sunburn. UVA rays have the ability to penetrate the skin more deeply, affecting the lower dermal layers, but do not significantly contribute to redness and sunburn. UVA has long been considered both the ageing and tanning ray. An easy way to remember this is UVA for *ageing;* UVB for *burning.* Both ultimately damage your skin, and so not too surprisingly we need protection against both.

HOW DOES UV LIGHT FROM THE SUN
CAUSE SKIN AGEING?

UV light causes damage to the skin via a number of molecular mechanisms. We still have a lot to learn in this field but research is providing more answers and therefore driving our skincare choices.

About 50 per cent of UV damage is from its causing the formation of free radicals, which are harmful to skin cells. The rest of the damage is from UV light causing direct cell injury and DNA damage. UV light has been shown to activate enzymes known as matrix metalloproteinases; these break down collagen and damage the skin's support structure, making it sag or deepening wrinkles. These enzymes also have the ability to prevent new collagen production. What you will see in the mirror as a result of these processes is sagging, wrinkles and thin, inelastic skin – the kinds of things we typically associate with ageing. Research also suggests that UV light causes accumulation of a protein known as progerin. This can limit the lifespan of skin cells and their ability to regenerate; the skin is therefore less effective in protecting us.

None of this spells good news for our skin. However, it is within our control to limit the amount of UV light to which our skin is exposed. Preventing damage is often more cost-effective than treatments trying to reverse the visible signs of ageing. If we think about it in these terms, why spend thousands of pounds undergoing invasive procedures to correct skin damage when you could spend under £20 on sunscreen to prevent the damage in the first place? In this day and age, focus should always be on preventative healthcare where possible.

There are factors other than sunshine that also contribute to external ageing to a lesser degree. These include smoking, diet and pollution. Collectively, these non-genetic, environmental factors are sometimes referred to as the 'exposome', and are discussed later in the book in chapter 6, 'Lifestyle'.

SKIN OF COLOUR

There are some important differences in skin of colour or ethnic skin. The pigment melanin, which gives our skin its colour, is present in higher quantities in those with dark skin. Melanin absorbs UV light and has the ability to block free radical damage. Darker skin is therefore relatively more protected from sun damage and ageing. Research suggests that black skin has a natural sun protection factor (SPF) of 13.4 compared to white skin, which is about 3.4.

Skin of colour develops problems with pigmentation more readily than white skin types. Inflammatory skin conditions such as acne, eczema and psoriasis can often leave dark staining in the skin that can persist for months. This is known as post-inflammatory hyperpigmentation.

The onset of wrinkles, skin laxity and sagging is less common in dark skin when compared to an age-equivalent individual with white skin. Despite this, even dark skin types are vulnerable to sun damage, just not to the same degree. Prolonged, cumulative sun exposure, however, will still lead to the signs we associate with ageing skin so those with dark skin types should also be practising preventative measures.

2

REGULAR SKINCARE

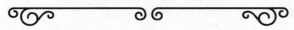

One thing that often comes up during my skin consultations is the confusion that lies around a regular skincare routine. Much of what we initially learn is passed down to us or simply observed behaviour we imitate from the older females in our lives. As we age, much of our advice is taken from popular culture, magazines and friends. Advice can often be conflicting, leaving you more baffled about the basics than before you started.

And that's just a problem for the women. Men often get taught even less about their basic skincare routine. There have been numerous situations in my clinic where I have had to explain, step-by-step, how to use a face wash or moisturizer to a teenage boy. This is through no fault of their own, but simply that no one has ever shown them how to do it.

Women can often fall into two camps when it comes to skincare. The first is guilty of having the same routine over the years despite seasonal or major life changes. There is a reluctance to switch it up and explore new ways of achieving the same end. The other gang is the skincare junkies – they love new beauty fads, products and complex, layering routines borrowed from our Korean cousins. Probably the best approach is somewhere in between, as all most of us want is an effective skincare routine that ideally takes the least amount of time to apply. We are a time-poor generation looking for instant results.

CLEANSING

A good cleansing routine is vital for keeping your skin healthy and preventing disease. It is worthwhile to get into good habits from an early age.

One of the main functions of skin is to act as a barrier to the outside world. The skin's barrier function can easily be disrupted or damaged by noxious chemicals such as pollutants in the environment, cumulative sun damage or even products that are deliberately applied to the skin for their anti-ageing effects, such as retinoids. Using a cleanser will not only remove all the grime we come into contact with as we're going about our daily business, from home to work to gym to bar. It also eliminates the micro-organisms with which we share our world and potentially improves the barrier function of the skin. This will give the natural glow of your skin the chance to really shine through.

Cleansing – and soap in particular – has a very long pedigree in human history. Cleansing was documented in the Ebers Papyrus, written in Ancient Egypt in around 1550 BC. The Egyptians wore heavy face make-up and used cleansing bars made from animal fat and perfume. In this day and age, we are spoilt for choice. We tend to take more care with the cleaning and maintenance of our face than we do the rest of our body, and as such, cleansing technology has developed to keep up with this. There is a wide range of cleansing products on the market. Facial cleansers include bar soaps, foaming and non-foaming cleansers, cleansing milks, toners, scrubs, micellar waters and oils. The choice is huge and the best product for you very much depends on your skin type, personal preference and budget.

There is a common misconception that expensive products work better than their cheaper counterparts. More often than not, this is not the case and the extra pennies are going into pretty packaging and clever marketing.

Bar soaps

Bar soaps can often be harsh for delicate facial skin and have the ability to interfere with normal skin function. They can strip out fats or lipids in the upper layer, affecting the skin's barrier. If the barrier is compromised, water loss through the skin is accelerated, leading to dryness. For most people, it is best to avoid these for facial cleansing. Those with oily skin types should be fine using them from time to time, but should probably not make a habit of it!

Foaming and non-foaming cleansers

Foaming or lathering cleansers are good for oily or blemish-prone skin types. The product is mixed with water and lathers up when wet. Non-foaming cleansers are a milder alternative and do not lather when mixed with water. They are helpful for dry or sensitive skin types. Their main problem is that they can leave a residue on the skin and many people feel their skin has not been cleansed thoroughly as a result.

Cleansing milks and toners

Cleansing milks and toners are used to cleanse with a cotton pad rather than using water. Cleansing milks dissolve oil and dirt and are suitable for dry skin. They can leave moisturizing agents on the skin which improve symptoms of dryness. Toners have had much popularity over the years and are often used to clean the skin and reduce apparent pore size. Toners are usually alcohol-based and can be used on oily or acne-prone skin. They are usually used after cleansing rather than as a stand-alone product. The alcohol content can sometimes result in dryness and irritation so should be used with caution.

Micellar waters

Micellar waters have been on the cleansing circuit for some time now. They use tiny micelles (small balls of cleansing-oil molecules) suspended in water to draw out skin impurities. They can be useful for all skin types but my feeling remains that they are most useful as a cleansing option when there is no water available. To use these as a primary cleanser after removing make-up and sunscreen at the end of the day requires a lot of time and product. They can, however, be useful as a second cleanse to remove any excess grime after the main cleanse has been carried out with another product.

Facial oils

Facial oils have gained much notoriety in recent years. They are touted as being good for all skin types – oily skin included. The theory is that 'like dissolves like' and, therefore, oil will dissolve oil. I have seen little evidence to back up the claim that facial oil is good for those of us prone to spots and my advice would be to steer clear of these unless you have dry or very dry skin. Oils on the skin can promote the formation of blackheads, leading to spots.

The Five Rules of Cleansing

---

1. Cleanse your face both morning and night. The evening cleanse is particularly important to remove make-up, sunscreen and particles of pollution we have come into contact with during the day. Failing to do this can result in breakouts, blemishes and potentially even premature skin ageing.

2. Face wipes are always a no-no unless you're using them as a last resort at the gym or on the go. This is because they can cause skin irritation, and mainly just smear dirt, make-up and oils across the skin's surface – you don't end up with a thorough cleanse.

3. If using water, the temperature should always be warm to lukewarm. Avoid using very hot or cold water – cold water is less effective at removing oils from the skin and hot water can leave the skin dry and irritated.

4. Never, ever apply a facial cleansing product directly to dry skin. It can lead to sensitivity.

5. Always use a towel to pat the face dry. Do not vigorously rub the skin as you dry it as this can lead to unnecessary irritation.

Double cleansing

The concept of double cleansing has become more common in recent years. For the more cynically minded, it is yet another beauty fad invented to make us part with our hard-earned cash. Double cleansing in the traditional sense involves the use of two different cleansers. The first cleanse is to remove make-up and SPF and the second is to clean more deeply and ensure any residue has been removed. Many people will recommend an oil-based cleanser followed by a foaming cleanser.

In actual fact, as with most things, it is difficult to be so prescriptive. For many people (e.g. those with acne or blemish-prone skin), I would recommend staying away from an oil cleanser; a micellar water may be more appropriate. For those with dry or sensitive skin, double cleansing may result in 'over-cleansing' and irritation. Choosing the right products for your skin type is absolutely vital but common sense is also needed. Double cleansing can be useful at night to remove heavy make-up but may be unnecessary otherwise.

Many people already double cleanse without realizing it. If you use make-up remover followed by a foaming wash, that is still an example of a double cleanse. In its most basic form, it simply means you are cleaning the skin twice.

The benefits of double cleansing are ensuring the skin is completely clear of make-up, SPF and other skincare products layered during the day. Further, it prepares the skin for any other topical treatments that are used afterwards.

SERUMS

Serums have been circulating the beauty and dermatology world for several years now. They are the next step in your skincare and should be used after cleansing and before moisturizing.

You can be entirely forgiven if you are uncertain about what they are and what they do! Many Western beauty products are derived from Korean skincare and their amazing (but time-consuming) multi-step rituals. Serums and, more recently, essences are ubiquitous in department stores.

Facial serums are concentrated, clear, gel-like solutions applied to the skin which consist of small molecules. This means that they are absorbed quickly and penetrate deep into the skin. This contrasts with a moisturizer, which has larger particles and is designed to hydrate the skin surface.

Serums are usually water-based. They do not contain occlusive, moisturizing ingredients such as petrolatum or mineral oil. They have a high concentration of active ingredients such as antioxidants, vitamins, peptides and brightening agents.

Serums can be used to treat a multitude of sins including dryness, fine lines, wrinkles, dark spots, uneven skin tone and premature skin ageing.

Serums are, generally speaking, good for all skin types. Your choice of serum depends very much on the skin concern you are trying to address:

- *Anti-ageing:* Antioxidant serums (e.g. those containing vitamin C, ferulic acid, resveratrol) can be particularly useful on a daily basis if anti-ageing is a concern.
- *Dry skin:* Hydrating serums with hyaluronic acid or vitamin E are good.
- *Oily skin:* These types can benefit from vitamin C and niacinamide.

Essences

Essences are now also commonly available in the Western world. They were borrowed from the Far East where they have been used for decades. Essences and serums are very similar. They both contain active ingredients but essences tend to be more watery in consistency. Do you need to use both? Probably not. Much of it has become about marketing. Stick to a serum and you should be fine.

Serums and essences usually tend to be relatively expensive due to their quantity of active ingredients. As they are concentrated, only a few drops or a dollop less than the size of a pea should be required. Use your fingertips to apply and press the serum or essence into the skin. Let it fully absorb and wait at least five minutes before going on to the next step – moisturizing.

MOISTURIZING

Moisturizer is necessary to maintain the elasticity and flexibility of the skin's upper layers. This keeps the skin healthy and allows it to function effectively as a barrier. The face is rarely covered and continuously exposed to the elements. Moisturizers can improve the texture or quality of skin, treat dryness and provide sun protection. There is plenty of scientific evidence to support their use. I have heard some odd claims in the media of moisturizers making your skin 'lazy' and less able to hydrate itself, but I can't say there is any robust data to back this up.

Moisturizer ingredients fall into three main categories: humectants, occlusives and emollients. Knowing what these do and what ingredients to look out for can help you choose the right one.

Humectants

Humectants are key in maintaining skin hydration; they act by attracting and chemically binding water in the skin. They have the ability to temporarily plump the skin and improve fine lines and wrinkles. Hyaluronic acid is a common agent used in skincare which functions as a humectant – it has the ability to bind 1,000 times its own weight in water. Other humectants include glycerine, hexanediol, butylene glycol and sorbitol.

One of the problems with humectants is that they extract water from the deeper skin layers to replenish the upper layer (the stratum corneum). Over time, they actually have the potential to cause greater dryness. The formulations tend to be light and are popular choices for the summer months but in the winter or in a very dry climate, occlusive moisturizers may be better for some. Glycerine, however, still remains one of the best ingredients in a moisturizer.

Occlusives

Occlusive agents create a barrier over the skin and prevent water loss from the surface. Occlusive products commonly include one or more of the following ingredients: dimethicone, squalene, propylene glycol, lecithin, cocoa butter, shea butter, lanolin, petrolatum, paraffin and beeswax. These are good for dry to very dry skin but often have a greasy, shiny finish and are cosmetically less acceptable. Newer agents can limit this but occlusive moisturizers should be avoided in those with oily or acne-prone skin.

Emollients

These are the third group of agents commonly found in moisturizers. Emollients include dimethicone, trisiloxane, ceramides, linoleic acid and caprylyl glycol to name a few. These act by replacing skin lipids and filling in the gaps or crevices between skin cells.

Many moisturizers actually contain a combination of humectants, occlusives and emollients. Some ingredients also have more than one function and can act simultaneously as an emollient and occlusive (e.g. dimethicone). In general terms, if your skin is acne prone you should go for products that are higher in humectants but low in occlusive agents. Conversely, if your skin is dry, a moisturizer with a higher content of emollients and occlusives will be better.

EYE CREAMS

The skin around the eyes is thin and delicate compared to the rest of our facial skin. The eye area is also extremely active – we blink on average more than 20,000 times a day! Skin at this site is fragile and needs to be looked after appropriately. I commonly get asked in clinic – and also by friends and family – about eye-specific concerns, and suitable products to use in this area.

Many facial moisturizers are suitable to use around the under-eye area and you do not necessarily need a separate product, contrary to popular belief. Generally speaking, if a product is suitable for the face, it should be fine to use around the eyes. If you look at the ingredients, there is no real difference between products for the eyes compared to the rest of the face. The main exceptions to this are if you suffer with oily skin and your regular day moisturizer is being used to combat this. Products made for blemish-prone skin may irritate and unnecessarily dry the under-eye area.

No amount of eye cream will improve age-related sagging or puffy eyes regardless of what the product promises you. The skin around the eyes is vulnerable to damage from the sun's radiation and whilst an eye cream will moisturize, plump the skin and temporarily improve fine lines, wearing SPF around the eyes is absolutely vital, if premature ageing is a concern.

Due to the sensitive nature of eyelid skin, care should be taken when applying eye cream. In particular, it is important not to pull or stretch the skin. Use a small pea-sized amount for each eye and either tap or massage your eye cream on your upper and lower eyelids. Do not use more product than necessary, as there is a chance it can get into the eyes and cause irritation. Wait a few minutes before applying make-up to ensure the product is fully dry and absorbed into the skin.

EXFOLIATION

Exfoliation should be a regular part of your skincare routine. It gives an instant improvement to the appearance of skin by removing the dull, dry layer of upper skin cells. Superficial exfoliation will not only make the texture of the skin look better, but will also improve age spots and uneven skin tone, as well as allowing better penetration of your serum or moisturizer. The long-term benefits, however, will only really be gained if exfoliation is carried out regularly as the treatment itself only affects the superficial top layer of cells. These are continually shed and replaced.

Exfoliation can either be mechanical or chemical. Mechanical exfoliators include sponges, facial brushes, scrubs and electronic cleansing devices. Devices, in particular, are highly efficient in hard-to-reach areas such as the sides of the nose. Scrubs containing sugar, crystals, sands and other rough particles can also effectively be used to unblock pores, reduce blackheads and remove dead, dull skin.

Chemical exfoliators use chemicals – usually acids – to dissolve dry skin cells. This isn't as awful as it sounds; the top layer of skin cells is already dead, and this process should never be painful! Once the exfoliating chemicals are removed, your skin should appear brighter and feel smooth. When you're in the skincare aisle, take a look at the ingredients label and keep an eye out for alpha-hydroxy acids (AHAs) and beta-hydroxy acids (BHAs). You may be familiar with these terms as they frequently appear in the popular beauty press, but there seems to be a bit of confusion about what they are and what they do.

AHAs are a group of natural acids often found in food and commonly used agents in skincare include glycolic acid (found in sugar cane), lactic acid (from milk) and malic acid (found in fruit, especially apples), although there are others. They work by breaking down the 'glue' that holds together surface skin cells. Glycolic acid also has extra benefits and with continued use will help fine lines, wrinkles and oily skin. For best results, choose skincare products that can be left on overnight (e.g. Pixi Glow Tonic or Peter Thomas Roth Glycolic Acid 10% Toning Complex).

BHAs are oil-soluble molecules that can penetrate into the pores rather than act on a superficial level. The most common BHA used in skincare is salicylic acid from willow bark. It has anti-inflammatory and antibacterial properties, so is a good choice for those with oily or blemish-prone skin. It must not be used during pregnancy, however, or if there is a known allergy to aspirin.

Both chemical and physical exfoliation can be effective and the preferred method is largely dependent on how sensitive an individual's skin is to the product being used. Those with rosacea or sensitive skin may find some of the chemical agents irritating to the skin. As such, they should be used with caution to see how their skin responds, and if tolerated then the frequency of usage may be gradually increased over days or weeks.

How often you need to exfoliate very much depends on your skin type. Those with oily skin find they can tolerate using an exfoliating agent daily whilst others with dry or sensitive skin may only manage once weekly or even less frequently. You may need to experiment with your skin to see what it will tolerate without dryness, or a burning or stinging sensation.

One of the most common errors in those with acne or oily skin is over-exfoliation in an attempt to unblock pores and remove oil. This is not a good idea, as exfoliating frequently with harsh agents will cause irritation and potentially a worsening of break-outs. The skin can end up sore, inflamed and irritated, but the acne will remain. If you find yourself in this situation, you may need to see a medical professional for help with your skin.

That said, AHAs and BHAs remain hero products of skincare and nearly all of us can benefit from incorporating them into our skincare regime. As they are effectively stripping away the upper layers of skin cells, however, they can make your skin more sensitive to sunshine; using sunscreen is therefore essential.

MASKS

Now, I love a mask as much as the next person, but sadly there is actually very little scientific evidence to prove that using face masks is of any real benefit to the skin's health in the long term. Most of our information on their use comes from the beauty industry itself, celebrity endorsement and anecdotal evidence.

That said, the mere process of spending some time spoiling oneself and investing in self-care is likely to have positive benefits to your stress levels and general health and well-being. For many, stress can lead to problem skin, so any method of combatting this can only be a good thing.

Face masks can be incorporated into your skincare routine at your convenience. Rather than buying into the name or a brand, again, the key is to look at ingredients to decide what is suitable for you. Oily skin will benefit from masks with clay, charcoal, witch hazel, salicylic acid, glycolic acid, niacinamide and tea tree oil to name a few. Sheet masks or masks with hyaluronic acid are generally good for dry or dehydrated skin that needs a boost. Sheet masks are easily portable and can be a treat for the skin following long-haul air travel after your skin has been subjected to recirculated air for many hours. Brightening masks with vitamin C can help lacklustre skin.

There is no harm in using masks regularly for your skin provided you choose what is right for you – a product that does not cause redness, irritation, peeling or sensitivity. However, the benefits are likely to be temporary and short-lived. From a pampering point of view though, highly recommended!

SUNSCREEN

This is the one universal item that every dermatologist worth their salt will agree needs to be part of your daily skincare routine. Sunscreen protects against solar radiation, in particular UVA and UVB. There are other forms of radiation, including infrared and high-energy visible light, and some sunscreens will also provide additional protection against these.

I frequently get asked whether it is necessary to have a regular SPF in the winter or if it is cloudy. The answer is always a loud and resounding 100 per cent YES. There is still ultraviolet radiation from the sun around in the winter when the days are shorter (albeit less) AND up to 80 per cent of ultraviolet light penetrates cloud cover.

Sunscreen has two main benefits, both of which are important. Firstly, sunscreen use will reduce your risk of skin cancer. Secondly, the sun's rays are responsible for about 80 to 90 per cent of the features we associate with ageing – fine lines, wrinkles, loss of skin elasticity and pigmentation. Sunscreen is your best protection against premature skin ageing in a bottle. Nothing else even comes close.

When looking for a good sunscreen for your face, choose a minimum of SPF 15–30 with UVA cover (it should say on the product). SPF 15 is fine for those with olive or darker skin types and SPF 30 for most white, Caucasian skin. Very fair pale skin could benefit from increasing the SPF to 50. Many cosmetic products such as moisturizer and foundation have SPF added to them and there is often confusion about whether this is enough or an extra sunscreen should also be used. The truth is that most of us do not use enough of our cosmetic product to achieve the same SPF as a sunscreen alone. In general terms, living in the UK as I do, using make-up with SPF when the days are short in the winter is probably fine. Due to our latitude, we get very little UVB between October and March – this is the sun's ray often associated with burning. In the spring and summer, however, it is worthwhile switching to a separate sunscreen to be used after your regular moisturizer.

However, this isn't a case of one size fits all and some common sense also needs to be employed. For example, if you are regularly using exfoliating products during the winter such as AHAs and BHAs, you are better off with a separate regular sunscreen. Similarly, if you participate in outdoor sports or work and are likely to be outside for longer than twenty minutes or so at a time you should wear daily sun protection. The same applies if you live in a sunny climate or close to the equator: wearing a regular daily sunscreen throughout the year is strongly advised.

For many, there is still a lack of clarity on what exactly SPF and its numerical value means. SPF or sun protection factor is only a measure of the ability of a sunscreen to protect against UVB radiation. UVB damages the skin's outer layers, contributing to sunburn. The SPF is a theoretical multiplier of the amount of time you can stay in the sun without getting burnt. So if your unprotected skin starts to go red after ten minutes in the sun, an SPF 20 will theoretically allow you to stay outdoors for 200 minutes (i.e. twenty times the original duration). In truth, this isn't necessarily that accurate as sunscreen is only one element of looking after your skin, many apply less than the correct amount and other factors such as distance from the equator, altitude and time of year will also have a part to play.

With all that in mind, then, using an SPF 30 will not provide twice as much protection as using SPF 15. Similarly, a factor 20 is not twice as good as a factor 10. An SPF 15 blocks about 93 per cent of UVB, SPF 30 blocks 97 per cent and SPF 50 blocks 98 per cent. So you can see there is actually very little difference between an SPF 30 and 50. There is no sunscreen that gives 100 per cent protection against the sun.

The SPF gives no indication whether a sunscreen is also offering you protection against UVA. UVA rays penetrate the skin deeper than UVB and are traditionally associated with ageing of the skin. Sunscreens sold in the EU have a 'star rating' for UVA or 'UVA logo' on the label. Most modern-day sunscreens are broad-spectrum which means they will provide protection against both UVA and UVB.

In the UK, whilst UVB levels fluctuate with the seasons, UVA remains relatively static through the year. UVA will also penetrate window glass. So if you work near a window or spend long periods of time driving, it is definitely worthwhile wearing sunscreen all year.

Choosing the correct sunscreen for your skin largely comes down to personal preference. Different types of sunscreen are discussed elsewhere but the key is to choose a formulation you feel happy with. Oily skin types should go for sunscreens with a matte finish and light gel or fluid textures, whereas those with dry skin can use rich creams and balms. Sensitive skin types might find that sunscreens with titanium dioxide and zinc oxide are better than those with chemical filters.

Sunscreen often comes in a moisturizing base and those with oily skin may not need to layer a moisturizer and sunscreen – the sunscreen alone may be sufficient. Sunscreen is the last skincare product applied before make-up. You should use about half a teaspoon of product to your face and neck. This needs to dry for three to five minutes before applying foundation.

Sunscreen Top Tips

- Daily sunscreen use can help guard against skin cancer and premature skin ageing.

- Choose a broad-spectrum sunscreen which offers protection against both UVA and UVB light.

- Sunscreen should be a minimum of SPF 15–30.

- Oily skin types should go for mattifying gels or fluid textures; dry skin types will benefit from rich creams and balms.

- Where possible it is better to wear a separate sunscreen rather than opt for cosmetic products that already contain SPF.

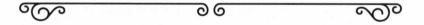

SKINCARE JARGON

How often do you walk down the skincare aisle and see products labelled as 'hypoallergenic' or 'dermatologically tested' or 'clinically proven' to do X, Y or Z? There is much beauty jargon and very few of us actually know what the fancy terms on product packaging mean. There is absolutely no doubt that the skincare industry takes complete advantage of this and, sadly, much of what we see is clever marketing. It is there to impress, baffle and mislead in equal measures as you hand over your money. So let's take a look at some common product labelling and what it really means.

Hypoallergenic

This is a manufacturer claim that a product will cause fewer allergies than others. It is not, however, a legally binding term: there is no minimum industry standard to prove the product causes fewer allergic reactions. It is there simply to imply to the consumer that the product will not cause irritation.

Unfortunately, there is no guarantee of this and the term is rather meaningless. Hypoallergenic products can still contain fragrances – a common cause of allergy and irritation. If you suspect you have an allergy to one of your personal care products, I'd advise you to see a dermatologist for formal allergy testing.

Non-comedogenic

This literally means 'will not block pores' and is often found on the label of skincare for those with acne or oily skin. If an ingredient is comedogenic, it will encourage blocked pores and the formation of blackheads.

Traditional gold-standard testing for comedogenicity was carried out on rabbit ears. Chemical ingredients were simply applied to the rabbit ears and scientists would look to see if comedones or blackheads developed. Although this method was commonly used, many cosmetic scientists and dermatologists felt it was inaccurate and misleading and many influential dermatologists later discredited its use. The EU has now banned animal testing and comedogenicity tests commonly take place on humans. Test ingredients are usually applied to the backs of human volunteers under occlusion for several weeks. Skin samples are then taken and analysed for blackheads.

The main problem with products labelled as 'non-comedogenic' is that, yet again, there are no industry standards or regulation. Generally speaking, those prone to breaking out are still better off looking for a light-textured non-comedogenic product BUT be aware that, despite the label, it can still clog pores.

Clinically proven

Often seen on products, usually in the anti-ageing sector, to make them sound like they have undergone rigorous scientific testing to prove they work. In truth, it is more deceptive marketing. 'Clinically proven' usually just means that a product was tried on a small number of people, with them subsequently reporting back their findings at the end of a set period of time. It is almost never a robust clinical trial with sound scientific methodology, an adequate sample size or appropriate statistical analysis. Unfortunately, short of contacting the manufacturer to request the original clinical data and then critically and scientifically appraising it, there is no way to be certain.

Dermatologically tested

Another term deliberately meant to lead you astray. It implies that the product has the endorsement of, or has passed rigorous laboratory tests carried out by, a dermatologist. In the UK, there is no legal definition of the term. According to EU guidance, the implication is that a dermatologist has supervised the testing on humans. However, there are no standard tests for the safety or efficacy of cosmetic products. This test could be as basic as a dermatologist or other qualified medical doctor giving the product to a handful of people to try and relaying back that there were no reports it caused irritation.

Natural

Natural skincare is another total minefield. Some have suggested that 'natural' should mean that at least 5 per cent or more of the ingredients are found in nature. Its definition, however, is not regulated in the US or UK, which again means there is no minimum standard for a product to qualify. There are a number of certification bodies that exist, each with some subtle differences (e.g. ECOCERT, NATRUE, The Soil Association and, more recently, the COSMOS standard).

The biggest difficulty is the lack of a standard definition: 'natural' can mean different things to different people. To me it might mean sourced from plants; to you it may mean that synthetic (i.e. man-made) ingredients are absent; to someone else natural skincare is that which is preservative free. You can see where the problems are going to arise with such a subjective term. To complicate things further, the original ingredient may be 'natural' (e.g. sourced from a flower or fruit), but chemical processing changes it from its original form to something quite different – is it then still 'natural'? Things to think about when you next reach for your natural skincare. The biggest mistake I see is that people equate natural skincare with somehow being safer than products lacking the label. Botanicals, herbs and essential oils can still cause irritation and allergies and these are commonly documented in scientific literature. People usually do not want to hear this but 'natural', in skincare, genuinely means very little.

Organic

The organic label in skincare is also not legally regulated in the UK – so the same issues around minimum standards and the exact definition still apply. It loosely means a product with ingredients that are grown without the use of artificial chemicals. The majority of these types of products that are certified organic often have non-organic ingredients also. As there is no legal definition and the various certification bodies have different criteria to meet for product labelling, there is no beauty industry standard. For example, depending on the organization, certain synthetic preservatives, hydrogenated oils and foaming agents may be permitted.

Things are a bit better in the US, where the USDA (United States Department of Agriculture) provides guidelines for organic labelling in cosmetics. For a product to be labelled 'organic', 95 per cent of its ingredients must be certified; 'organic-derived' products need only contain 70 per cent.

My advice would be to look at the label and then look at the ingredients. These are listed in descending order of their percentage of a product's composition. If the top three to five ingredients are synthetic (in general, if they have long, unpronounceable chemical names, you can be confident they're synthetic), it may not be an appropriate choice if you want genuine 'organic' skincare. But a word of caution that processing methods, additives and simply the ingredients themselves still have the ability to cause skin irritation and allergy.

There is a growing notion that natural and organic products are somehow better for you and safer for your skin. This is not true, and is simply the product of marketing and scaremongering. Just because a product comes from a plant does not make it safe. The incredibly toxic belladonna, also known as deadly nightshade, is testament to this.

For some, it is more the concern about having products with ingredients that are pesticide-free. There is, however, little evidence to show that pesticides in skincare products can penetrate the skin barrier. In fact, purifying and processing methods during the production process are likely to remove any pesticide traces that may remain on the raw ingredients.

Organic and natural skincare products are a choice. Some will still prefer to use these as they feel like a healthier lifestyle option, and that's okay. But remain mindful that they may not be any better for your skin. The label itself may not be the halo you first took it for.

Fragrance free

Fragrance free should mean exactly what it says on the tin but this is not always the case. The only way to be entirely certain that a product is really fragrance free is to check the ingredients list. Fragrance can cause allergies in susceptible individuals and irritation in those with sensitive skin. It is often marked as 'parfum' or 'fragrance' and is usually a blend of many agents. In the EU, there are twenty-six additional fragrance ingredients that by law also need to be declared separately from these if their concentration is above 0.001 per cent for products left on the skin (e.g. moisturizers, sunscreen), and 0.01 per cent for those that are washed off (e.g. face wash, shampoo).

If your skin is sensitive to fragrance, or you otherwise choose to avoid it, these are the additional twenty-six ingredients to look out for:

- alpha-isomethyl ionone
- amyl cinnamal
- amyl cinnamyl alcohol
- anise alcohol
- benzyl alcohol
- benzyl benzoate
- benzyl cinnamate
- benzyl salicylate
- butylphenyl methylpropional
- cinnamal
- cinnamyl alcohol
- citral
- citronellol
- coumarin
- eugenol
- evernia furfuracea extract
- evernia prunastri extract
- farnesol
- geraniol
- hexyl cinnamal
- hydroxycitronellal
- hydroxyisohexyl-3-cyclohexene-carboxaldehyde

- isoeugenol
- limonene
- linaool
- methyl 2-octynoate

Also, remain cautious of essential oils in products that are not subject to these EU rules as they can have the same natural constituents that are used in fragrances. For example, 'natural' skincare containing clove oil is likely to have the fragrance isoeugenol (mentioned in the list above). This still has the ability to cause irritation or allergy, despite being a 'natural' ingredient. You need to do your homework if you don't want to get caught out.

Free from chemicals

Now, this one is definitely a label to ignore. Technically speaking, *everything* is made from chemicals – be they natural or man-made. It is simply impossible to have a product that is 100 per cent chemical free. What is actually more important is whether a product and its ingredients are safe. An ingredient is not, by virtue of being 'natural', automatically more likely to be safer than a synthetic – i.e. man-made – one. The key is the amount, dose or concentration of the ingredients that are used. The EU regulates the maximum safe amount or concentration of what is safe in skincare. The regulations – and cosmetic science on which these are based – are very complex, but the interested reader (preferably with a background in chemistry!) can find out more in the cosmetics section of the European Commission website.

Vegetarian/vegan

In the UK, there is no legally binding definition of a vegetarian or vegan product and you are very much relying on the manufacturer to not be making unsubstantiated claims. Organizations such as PETA provide a list of animal-derived ingredients to avoid; the Vegetarian Society has a number of approved products. It can be difficult to be entirely certain whether the manufacturing process uses animal-derived agents that do not appear in the final product.

Preservative free

There are few cosmetic products that are truly and completely preservative free, but do we really want them to be? Preservatives are an important component of skincare and are added to beauty products to enhance their shelf-life by preventing the growth of bacteria, yeast and mould. Clearly, this is a good thing (and it would be far worse not to have them); smearing germ-contaminated products around the face or near the eyes is likely to lead to infection.

If a product contains water (aqua), it is very likely it also has a preservative, without which it would go off in a matter of days. Common preservatives include:

a) Formaldehyde preservatives or releasers

Don't be alarmed to see formaldehyde-based ingredients used as preservatives! There is EU regulation restricting how much formaldehyde can be present in a skincare product, and such concentrations as are used in this context are considered safe.

Formaldehyde preservatives are popularly used in personal-care products as they are effective and relatively cheap, showing activity against bacteria and some viruses. Ingredients to look out for in this category include quaternium-15, DMDM hydantoin, diazolidinyl urea, imidazolidinyl urea and 2-bromo-2-nitropropane-1,3-diol.

b) Methylisothiazolinone (MI) / methylchloroisothiazolinone (MCI)

MI and MCI are 'broad-spectrum' preservatives, meaning they have activity against a range of microbes. These chemical agents hit the news some years ago as a cause of skin allergy in susceptible individuals. As a result, European regulation no longer allows these agents to be present in 'leave-on' cosmetics such as face creams and wet wipes; they are, however, still allowed in low concentrations in rinse-off products such as shower gels and shampoos, and are safe to use in this context.

c) Parabens

Parabens have been used as preservatives since the 1950s. Common parabens found in skincare include methylparaben, ethylparaben, propylparaben and butylparaben.

Preservatives have had a bit of a raw deal in the skincare press over recent years due to concerns about their safety, allergy and sensitivity. Parabens, in particular, hit the newsstands some years ago due to having a weak effect similar to the hormone

oestrogen. Concern was raised that parabens in deo-
dorants might contribute to breast cancer following
trace amounts noted in breast cancer tissue. The
relevant scientific study was later discredited. No
cause and effect was confirmed; the mere presence
of parabens does not mean they contributed to causing cancer. An independent review carried out by
the European Commission in 2005 reiterated this.
There are strict guidelines regarding paraben type,
dose and concentrations used in skincare to ensure a
minimum safety standard is met and evidence shows
they are safe.

d) Are 'natural' preservatives better than synthetic preservatives?

As the demand for 'natural' skincare grows, so does
the demand for 'natural' preservatives. As the popular media has demonized synthetic preservatives,
many consumers choose products with alternatives.
Some difficulties with natural preservatives are that
they often do not have the same anti-microbial activity as their synthetic counterparts. There are fewer
options, and high concentrations may be required
for the formulation to be effective, which in turn
may cause skin sensitivity over time. Variation can

also exist between product batches depending on how the product was grown and harvested.

Personally, I think it's an individual choice; I have little hesitation in using synthetic preservatives and would not by default opt for a 'natural' one. There is no scientific evidence that natural preservatives are safer than synthetic ones. At the risk of seeking controversy, I think the natural beauty industry capitalizes on people's fear of unknown ingredients coupled with the growing 'wellness' trend. Cosmetic science should be evidence-based and not simply encourage the idea that because an ingredient comes from Mother Earth, it is safe.

Final thoughts on skincare jargon

The best habit to get into when purchasing skincare products is to become more familiar with their ingredients and what they do. This is more important than the label put together for you by the branding and marketing team. This chapter hopefully provides a starting point for you to become more aware of what the small print on the labels means, and also silences some of the bafflement that the vague terms and long and impenetrable chemical names may induce!

What I would encourage you to ask yourself next time you're in the cosmetics aisle is whether spending £200 on a serum simply because it's 'dermatologically tested' is really worth it – or are the ingredients very similar to something that can be purchased for one tenth that price? The expensive product may look attractive in your bathroom cabinet, but is it really any better for your skin than the cheaper alternative? Not necessarily. And if you still have any doubt, see a cosmetic dermatologist who is able to guide you.

3

SKINCARE REGIMES

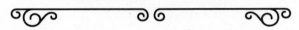

Most people will have skin types that fall into one of the following categories: oily, dry, sensitive, normal/combination. A person's skin type can change over time and skincare will also need to change in response to this.

OILY SKIN

Oily skin types often have visible pores, shiny or thick skin, and a predisposition to blackheads and other blemishes. It can change under the influence of weather and hormones.

This is one I can certainly relate to on a personal level, having had oily skin and the tendency to break out for most of my adult life. So for any of you suffering from bumpy, shiny skin and pores the size of planets, I'm right there with you.

But fear not! Here's an example skincare plan for oily skin:

AM routine

- Cleanse
- Eye cream
- Antioxidant serum (if ageing is a concern)
- Moisturizer with SPF or sunscreen
- Make-up

PM routine

- Double cleanse
- Eye cream
- Spot treatments, if needed (e.g. retinoid)
- No need for night cream unless skin is dry or tight

Consider exfoliation once or twice per week.

DRY SKIN

At the other end of the spectrum from oily skin, another very common issue is dry skin. This brings its own set of woes, but also specific ways of successfully managing them.

With dry skin, there is a tendency towards redness, scaly patches and the feeling of tightness. Pore size is very small but there are visible lines and the skin can be rough, itchy or flaky, and feel irritated. It is often worse in the winter months as it is aggravated by cold and windy weather conditions. This is also the time of year when we switch on the central heating, which further zaps the moisture from our skin. Furthermore, skin can become drier with age, particularly after the menopause.

If you do have dry skin, it needs to be looked after carefully. Avoid long, hot showers that can strip the skin further of moisture. Use gentle soaps and cleansers and avoid unnecessary exfoliation, which will only lead to further irritation. Scrubs, wash cloths and other cleansing devices can potentially aggravate dryness. Opt for rich-textured moisturizers or ointments and use as often as necessary to keep your skin feeling soft and supple.

An example skincare plan for dry skin:

AM routine

- Cleanse
- Eye cream
- Hydrating antioxidant serum
- Moisturizer
- Sunscreen
- Make-up

PM routine

- Cleanse
- Eye cream
- Moisturizer

Dry skin can benefit in the short-term from hydrating masks but exfoliation should be carried out with caution once or twice a month if tolerated.

SENSITIVE SKIN

Interestingly, there is no fixed dermatological definition of sensitive skin; it depends on how the individual reports the sensations of their skin. It is definitely a recognized skin type characterized by facial redness, burning, itching and dryness to varying degrees.

It is always worth seeking advice from a dermatologist when it comes to facial redness and skin sensitivity, particularly if this is an ongoing issue. There are many possible medical reasons for sensitive skin (e.g. rosacea and eczema) in addition to allergies to products that you may be applying. A dermatologist will be able either to diagnose and treat, or to exclude, these concerns. Despite this, there are many people with sensitive skin who do not have an obvious underlying skin disorder.

It is important for those with sensitive skin to try to identify their triggers and then avoid these as much as possible. It can be hard to manage, however, as skin sensitivity can often be unpredictable. Harsh soaps, toners and astringents should be avoided. Watch out for sodium lauryl sulphate, ammonium lauryl sulphate, salicylic acid, AHAs and alcohol. Fragrances can be a common culprit of irritation and the use of facial oils to combat dryness in this context can potentially make things worse. Opt for sunscreens with zinc or titanium (mineral-based sunscreens) rather than those with chemical filters that also have the potential to drive sensitivity.

An example skincare plan for sensitive skin:

AM routine

- Cleanse
- Eye cream
- Hydrating serum if dryness is a problem
- Moisturizer
- Sunscreen
- Make-up

PM routine

- Cleanse
- Eye cream
- Moisturizer if needed

Avoid exfoliating products as these can aggravate sensitive skin.

NORMAL/COMBINATION SKIN

Normal skin is that which, on the whole, has very few problems. It is not too oily and not too dry. There may, however, be a slightly oilier T-zone affecting the forehead, nose and chin.

An example skincare plan for normal/combination skin:

AM routine

- Cleanse
- Eye cream
- Antioxidant serum
- Moisturizer with SPF and/or sunscreen
- Make-up

PM routine

- Double cleanse
- Eye cream
- Moisturizer if needed

Exfoliation or applying face masks once a week can also provide benefit to this skin type without causing any problems with irritation.

4

HORMONES

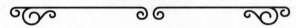

Skin concerns can often be attributed to hormonal changes that take place during the course of one's life. There are certain periods, namely puberty, pregnancy and the menopause, where this holds particularly true. Hormones can wreak havoc on the skin in a rather predictable manner during these times.

Hormones are chemical messengers that act on target bodily tissues. Skin changes are often related to fluctuation in the sex hormones – testosterone, oestrogen and, to a lesser degree, progesterone. These are produced in ovaries, testes and adrenal glands. Male hormones – in particular, testosterone – are sometimes known as androgens. Even women produce small quantities of androgens.

PUBERTY

The average age for a boy to begin puberty is twelve years and for girls it is eleven. By far the commonest skin problem encountered during puberty is acne, which is discussed in more detail in chapter 5. During this time, androgen levels begin to rise in both boys and girls. Raised androgen levels act on the skin's oil or sebaceous glands to make them bigger and start producing more sebum. This is one of the primary factors in the development of acne.

It is estimated that 85 per cent of teenagers will suffer from acne at some point to varying degrees of severity. During adolescence, acne is more common in males than females. Acne can strike any area in which there is a high density of oil-producing glands; the face, back and chest are commonly affected.

Teenagers with acne should be offered support as it is recognized that the condition can lead to altered body image and low self-esteem. This can often be overlooked by both family and health professionals alike. There are good over-the-counter and prescription medications to treat this condition and acne should never be dismissed as a cosmetic problem. Teens are often told they will 'grow out of it', almost as though acne is an insignificant phase or even some peculiar rite of passage. If it is severe, or mood-affecting, it should absolutely not be ignored and help should be sought. Having myself suffered between the ages of twelve and seventeen before finally going on a treatment that actually worked, starting university with clear skin was life-changing. I only wish I'd received the help I needed sooner and been more open about how my skin made me feel.

Aside from acne, raised androgen levels will also contribute to a number of other skin issues. These include increased sweating from the armpits, development of pubic and armpit hair, and an increase and darkening of moles on the body.

PREGNANCY

Pregnancy affects the skin due to physiological changes taking place in the body (e.g. increased blood flow) as well as hormonal changes. Increased blood flow can cause red palms (palmar erythema), dilated blood vessels (spider naevi and telangiectasia) and varicose veins. Hormonal changes can promote acne, stretch marks, melasma, hair loss, rashes and itching.

Acne

Acne in pregnancy is common and affects nearly 50 per cent of women. Increased levels of the hormone progesterone, usually in the first trimester, are to blame. Those with a previous history of acne are more likely to be affected but often things improve as pregnancy progresses.

Managing acne in pregnancy can be tricky, as most standard treatments should be avoided. It is always best to try and get your acne under control before pregnancy, but obviously that is often easier said than done. Over-the-counter preparations using glycolic acid can be helpful. Certain topical prescription agents such as azelaic acid and oral antibiotics like erythromycin, cephalexin and azithromycin are considered safe and pose no known risks to the baby. For the odd isolated large spot, steroid injections directly into the spot can be considered. Light therapies are also likely to be safe. These treatments are discussed further in chapter 5.

Acne in pregnancy can be managed but if problematic usually requires the input of a dermatologist to guide treatments safely and effectively.

Stretch marks

The dreaded stretch marks (striae gravidarum) are another skin change commonly associated with pregnancy, affecting nearly 80 per cent of women to some degree. Stretch marks usually affect the abdomen, thighs and breasts and start to develop after the sixth month of pregnancy. Very few people (i.e. those with very good genes!) escape completely unscathed.

Stretch marks develop not just due to the simple stretching of skin, but also because of hormonal changes associated with pregnancy. Pregnancy hormones cause a softening of the pelvic ligaments to allow for the delivery of the baby, but at the same time also soften skin fibres, which makes them more susceptible to stretching and tearing. Both these factors result in the development of stretch marks.

When they first develop, stretch marks are often pale pink in colour but can become very red or violaceous. Over time, the colour fades and the lines become silvery-white and wrinkled. Risk factors often quoted for developing stretch marks include a younger age at pregnancy, family history of stretch marks and pregnancy weight gain. These links have not been consistently reproducible in scientific studies.

Many products are promoted to prevent the development of stretch marks and women can end up spending a small fortune during pregnancy on skincare. Sadly, the scientific evidence-based answer suggests that topical treatments will not prevent their development, and this was indeed the conclusion of a large review in 2012. Not much has changed since then and large scientific trials with robust data are lacking. It is also not clear whether it is simply the action of massaging the skin (when rubbing the product in) that may help, more than the actual product being used. Really the best advice is to keep your skin well-moisturized during pregnancy but not fall into the trap of thinking that some magic (and no doubt expensive) cream will prevent stretch marks from forming.

Once stretch marks have formed, they can be difficult to treat. They can cause a great deal of distress and cosmetic concern and this is often wrongly dismissed. Whilst treatments are unlikely to get rid of them entirely, there are options which may improve the appearance to some degree. These include retinoid-based creams, micro-needling, radio-frequency devices and laser therapies; these are discussed in more detail in chapter 7, 'Anti-ageing Treatments'. It is worthwhile seeing an expert cosmetic dermatologist with experience in these treatments to choose the best option based on the severity of the stretch marks and your skin type.

Melasma

Melasma, sometimes known as chloasma or pregnancy mask, is skin discolouration than can develop for the first time during pregnancy. It often affects the forehead, cheeks and upper lip. The upper lip area, in particular, can create much anxiety, as women that are suffering feel it gives them the appearance of having a moustache, a comment I have heard very frequently in clinic. Hormonal changes that are not fully understood are thought to be responsible, in particular, fluctuations in oestrogen and melanocyte-stimulating hormone (MSH). Melasma brought on by pregnancy can fade after delivery but can return during subsequent pregnancies.

Melasma treatments are discussed in detail in chapter 5, 'Specific Skin Concerns'. During pregnancy, it is vital to wear sunscreen as sunlight can drive the melasma process. Most other recommended treatments should be avoided until the baby's birth.

Pigmentation

Pregnancy hormones, in particular MSH, are thought to play a role in skin darkening of the areolae and nipples. Linea nigra, often known as the pregnancy line, can also develop. This is a dark vertical line in the centre of the abdomen (from the umbilicus to the pubic bone) that usually becomes visible after the fifth month of pregnancy. It gradually fades after pregnancy.

Telogen effluvium

Telogen effluvium is temporary loss of hair from the scalp and is very common, affecting nearly 40 per cent of post-pregnancy women, usually in the first three months after delivery. This problem frequently comes to my attention in clinic as skin and hair are closely related, and hair falls within my remit as a consultant dermatologist. As it affects so many women after pregnancy, it deserves a specific call-out.

During pregnancy, higher levels of oestrogen and pro-gesterone keep hairs in their growth phase (known as 'anagen') and many women note their hair is thicker dur-ing this time. After delivery, hormone levels change rapidly to normal and this 'shock' is thought to switch hairs from the growth to the shedding phase (known as 'telogen'), resulting in hair falling out. The good news is that, like most changes associated with pregnancy, this is a temporary prob-lem which settles over six to twelve months.

Itchy skin

Itching that manifests without a rash is extremely common during pregnancy due to increased oestrogen levels. In addition, stretching of the skin, particularly in the latter half of pregnancy, can also cause itching.

General measures to alleviate this include taking cool baths and showers. Avoid harsh soaps and detergents on the skin and use mild, fragrance-free cleansers. Keep the skin well-hydrated and moisturized, and avoid getting too hot.

There is, in addition, an uncommon condition called cholestatic pruritus which can cause intractable itching and is associated with raised bile salts and liver enzymes. If your itching is unbearable or stopping you from sleeping it is worthwhile discussing this with your GP or antenatal team as you may require a blood test to look for this condition.

Specific pregnancy rashes

a) Pruritic urticated papules and plaques of pregnancy (PUPPP)

This one is a bit of a mouthful but is sometimes known by the slightly easier (but not much!) term 'polymorphic eruption of pregnancy'.

PUPPP usually develops in the third trimester and settles a few weeks after delivery. It consists of a rash which can look like a mixture of hives and red bumps or patches on the skin that often start on the abdomen, within stretch marks. This is usually extremely itchy and most often affects a first pregnancy. It can be associated with rapid or extreme weight gain or multiple pregnancies such as twins.

We do not know the exact cause of this condition, though there are a number of hypotheses for its onset. Treatment requires emollient washes, antihistamines and prescription steroid creams or ointments to reduce inflammation. The condition is uncomfortable but will not harm the baby.

b) Pemphigoid gestationis

This is a rare condition that can occur in pregnancy, which may be aggravated by raised oestrogen levels. It is an 'auto-immune' blistering disease – the mother's immune system goes into a state of overdrive and starts producing antibodies which attack her own skin. A blistering rash occurs in mid to late pregnancy (thirteen to forty weeks). Initially, this starts as an itchy rash, often around the umbilicus, appearing like hives or red bumps and patches. They can extend to involve the trunk and limbs. Within a week or two, tense blisters can develop containing clear fluid.

If pemphigoid gestationis is suspected, early input from a dermatologist is necessary; to confirm, they may carry out a biopsy, a surgical procedure in which a small piece of skin is removed and taken to the lab for testing. There is, with this condition, an increased risk of premature delivery and occasionally the newborn baby can also develop a blistering rash, which clears up at about six weeks. Pemphigoid gestationis requires treatment with steroid creams/tablets, together with antihistamines. Most women will find their symptoms improve towards the end of pregnancy but many get a flare-up of the rash at the time of delivery. This needs to be managed carefully with good communication between the obstetric team and dermatologists to coordinate the appropriate treatment.

MENOPAUSE

Skin problems are a big issue during the menopause. Women are living longer and average female life expectancy in the UK is now nearly eighty-three years. Interestingly, although life expectancy continues to rise, the average age of onset of menopause has changed relatively little over the past century. This means there are far more women suffering with skin issues associated with the menopause for a much longer period of time. For the beauty industry, this market is huge and will only continue to grow as standards of living and medical innovations improve.

In the run-up to the menopause, or 'perimenopausal' period, women will start to notice changes in their skin. This starts from approximately the mid-forties onwards, when oestrogen levels start to decline. For some women, this can lead to the development of acne. As oestrogen levels fall, androgen levels become proportionately more dominant, which can drive oil gland activity. Others, however, may start to notice dryness and red patches on the skin.

Once women reach the menopause and afterwards, the body goes into a relatively oestrogen-deficient state. Lack of oestrogen is the most common cause of post-menopausal skin issues. Common problems include:

Skin dryness

There is a reduction in skin metabolism. Skin functions less effectively as a barrier resulting in increased water loss. This will leave the skin vulnerable to the elements. Alongside this, there is reduced oil and lipid production in the skin. These factors acting together promote dryness, so the use of a rich, creamy moisturizer is key.

Wrinkles

After the menopause, women's skin thickness decreases by 1.13 per cent per year due to falling collagen levels. In the first five years after menopause, collagen content is thought to decrease by as much as 30 per cent. Collagen is much needed for the skin's support structure. Hormones and cumulative sun damage work in synchrony to promote wrinkles and sagging. Specific creams, injectable agents and laser treatments can counter these natural changes associated with ageing; as such, these strategies are discussed in detail in chapter 7, 'Anti-ageing Treatments'.

Increased fragility

As the skin thins with age, there is also loss of fat and connective tissue support around blood vessels, which makes them more susceptible to injury. Oestrogen has a protective role in wound healing and reduced levels of this after menopause mean that the skin takes longer to heal following trauma.

Redness/sensitive skin

Redness can occur due to hot flushes associated with the menopause. A skin condition known as rosacea can also develop for the first time leading to redness and sensitivity.

Facial hair

Straggly facial hair often starts to appear on the chin and upper lip. This again is due to a change in the ratio of oestrogen to androgen hormones in the bloodstream. Hairs can be tweezed, plucked, threaded or waxed, or removed with electrolysis or laser if they are dark.

Oestrogen is what keeps our hair and skin youthful. Hormone replacement therapy (HRT) may help maintain skin elasticity, moisture and thickness. However, not everyone is suitable for, or wants to take, HRT, and this decision needs to be made after discussion with your family doctor.

Phyto-oestrogens have gained popularity in recent years. These have a very similar chemical structure to oestrogen and can exert their effects in the body by binding to oestrogen receptors in cells. They can be found in dietary supplements or foods such as soy, yam, tofu and linseed. For some, it is seen as a more natural alternative to taking

HRT. However, there is still a lack of robust clinical trials to show whether they cause a significant increase in collagen production or what their long-term safety profile looks like. Most data at present is limited to laboratory or animal studies.

Getting skincare right after the menopause is important. Using a retinoid-based product at night will boost collagen production. An antioxidant serum will limit potential damage to already fragile skin. Many women will need to moisturize with rich creams on a daily basis due to dryness that can often set in during this period of life. Anti-ageing strategies are discussed in detail in chapter 7, 'Anti-ageing Treatments'.

Top Tips for Post-menopausal Skin

- Choose cream cleansers for dry skin rather than foaming washes.

- Hydrate the skin and moisturize with rich creams rather than gels morning and evening.

- Use a daily broad-spectrum SPF 15–30.

- Keep up with regular exercise to boost blood flow to the skin.

- Exfoliate regularly to keep a glowing complexion and help fade brown marks.

5

SPECIFIC SKIN CONCERNS

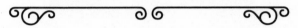

ACNE

Now this is a topic close to my own heart and the reason I ended up as a dermatologist. Stubborn, recalcitrant acne has plagued me for well over two decades and I know only too well the issues it can bring. Cancelled nights out, excessive use of make-up, anxiety that you may end up in a situation where someone will see your naked face. Simply just feeling ugly and ashamed. Even when your skin clears, the niggling fear persists that it may all return one day. And in my case, it usually does.

As a teenager, my skin problems caused a world of pain. I was about twelve years old when my acne started. Sadly it developed around the same time as my father's untimely death, which resulted in personal circumstances changing. In the space of a few short weeks, I was suddenly confronted with bereavement, a new school in an unfamiliar place and trying to make friends, all whilst having dreadful acne. I was painfully shy and it was hard. I didn't want people to look at me. All I could see in the mirror were my spots. My eye would not catch the normal skin between them. They disgusted me and I was certain that anyone who looked upon me would feel the same. Unsurprisingly, I didn't make many friends.

As an adult with acne, spots continue to evoke shame, embarrassment and feelings of inadequacy. It also generates anger: I should have grown out of this by now! In meetings, you wonder if others are taking you seriously, when inside you feel like a spotty teenager. Or, if your skin is bad enough, you cancel the meetings altogether for fear of being looked at or, worse still, judged. I know I am not alone in this. These are the same sentiments I hear being echoed by my patients in clinic on a daily basis. Acne can have profound effects on self-esteem and confidence.

The good news is that acne can be treated in a number of ways. No one should need to suffer. It is, however, important to seek advice early to prevent psychological and physical scarring, both of which can be much more difficult to manage than the acne itself.

What is acne?

Acne and 'spots' are the same thing. Acne is simply the medical term that doctors use.

Acne is increasingly being considered a chronic disease. This means that whilst it may be controlled, there might be no long-term cure: treatment can be successful but acne can recur over time. Coming to terms with this and realizing there is always a possibility it may come back is the first step to acceptance of this condition.

Acne is a disorder of the pilosebaceous unit of the skin. This consists of a hair follicle and its associated sebaceous or

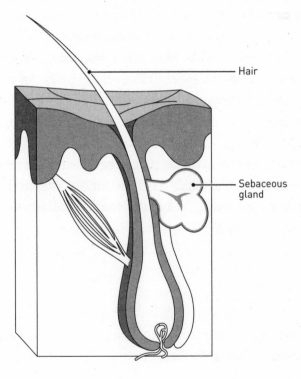

Hair

Sebaceous
gland

oil gland. Blockage or inflammation of the pilosebaceous units will result in acne. Oil glands are found in highest density on the face, back and chest and these are therefore the commonest sites of acne development.

What does acne look like?

Acne can manifest in a number of ways. It can be non-inflammatory and start as blackheads (open comedones) and whiteheads (closed comedones). These look like little bumps under the surface of the skin due to blocked pores. Over time, it can become more inflammatory and small red bumps (papules) or pus-filled spots can occur. In more severe forms, deep, red, tender spots known as nodules or cysts develop. This form – sometimes known as cystic acne – can result in scarring and needs more aggressive treatment. In practice, it is actually quite common for one person to have a variety of acne types (i.e. a combination of comedones and inflammatory spots).

Who gets acne?

Acne is one of the commonest skin problems and nearly everybody will suffer to some degree at some point during the course of their lifetime. In the UK, it accounts for more than 3.5 million GP appointments per year. It affects 80 per cent of people at some point between eleven and thirty years of age. During adolescence, acne is more common in males than females; this situation reverses in adulthood. It can also develop for the first time over the age of twenty-five, a scenario thought to affect up to 20 per cent of women and 8 per cent of men.

So whilst suffering from acne can feel very isolating, remember that almost everyone will struggle with it at some point. You're not facing this battle alone, so don't hesitate to seek medical advice or treatment if you need it!

What is the cause of acne?

Acne develops due to the complex interplay between a number of factors.

a) Puberty

As we hit puberty, our bodies start to produce male hormones known as androgens (in particular, the hormone testosterone). Women also produce androgens, albeit in smaller quantities than men. These androgens act on the oil glands, causing them to increase oil production. At the same time, cells lining the hair follicle become 'sticky' and start clumping together in a process known as follicular hyperkeratinization. The end result is that pores become blocked with sticky skin cells and excess oil. A bacterium known as *Propionibacterium acnes* (*P. acnes*), which lives on the skin, can then colonize these areas, stimulating inflammation and deeper spots.

b) Genetics

Genetics are thought to play an important role in the development of acne, mainly as the size and activity of the oil glands is inherited from our parents. Many people who suffer with acne are likely to have relatives that have also been affected during their lifetime (though this isn't always the case; I seem to be the only unlucky member of my family that suffers with spots!). Either way, don't be alarmed by the factors you can't control; there are always effective treatment options available.

c) Other causes

There are some other, less common, causes of acne, which include:

- cosmetics
- hair-styling products such as waxes or gels, which contain ingredients like lanolin, beeswax and petroleum jelly
- medications (e.g. corticosteroids, lithium, iodides)
- medical conditions that can cause hormonal fluctuations (e.g. polycystic ovarian syndrome, in which androgen levels are higher than usual)
- occlusion from wearing headbands, shoulder pads and backpacks

Does facial mapping for acne work?

Acne face mapping is an ancient practice derived from traditional Chinese medicine. People that support this practice report that the location of facial acne presents clues about what is causing it. For example, one such interpretation is that forehead spots are a result of diets high in processed food. I would stress that there is absolutely no scientific evidence for facial mapping and my strong recommendation would be to steer clear of anyone offering this type of advice. It preys on vulnerable people who are already having issues with their skin. You don't want to be caught out by these people who'll promise you the world and take your money but fail to deliver results. If you want to improve your acne, seek guidance and treatment from a properly trained medical professional, following the advice in this chapter to find the help you need.

Is it possible that acne in certain parts of the face may have an underlying cause?

Yes, it is. I expand on these below:

a) Forehead spots

Certain hair-styling products such as oils and waxes can cause forehead acne, particularly blackheads or whiteheads. The products themselves actually block pores, resulting in what is known as 'pomade acne'.

Forehead acne can also occur if you keep your hair in a fringe. Hair will rub against the forehead skin causing irritation and potentially contributing to breakouts (*acne mechanica*). The same applies to regularly wearing hats, caps and helmets. If your hair is oily, this may further aggravate the problem. The best way to solve this is to avoid wearing your hair in a fringe. If you absolutely can't be parted from your fringe, however, you might want to try limiting the time it sits against your forehead. You could also make simple changes such as wearing a headband at the gym or a shower cap when doing deep-conditioning hair treatments.

b) Lower cheek and jawline

This can be related to smartphone use, particularly when it is much worse on one side of your face. Touchscreens contain large numbers of bacteria on their surfaces. Placing your phone against your cheek creates pressure that may activate your sebaceous glands. Combined with heat generated from the phone and bacteria on the phone surface, acne can result. Get into the habit of cleaning your smartphone regularly, and where possible use hands-free.

In men, shaving and in-grown hairs can commonly cause acne or folliculitis (inflamed hair follicles) in the cheek, chin, jawline and neck area.

Why am I still getting acne in my thirties/forties?

The number of dermatology clinic visits for female adults over the age of twenty-five suffering with acne appears to have increased over the past decade. It is not entirely clear why this is the case.

Two distinct subtypes of adult female acne may be defined according to onset: 'persistent' and 'late-onset'. Persistent acne is that which develops in the teenage years and fails to spontaneously resolve by the third decade of life. Patients who suffer from persistent acne have spots intermittently or continuously during this time. They make up about 80 per cent of cases of female adult acne, and constitute the group of women that simply do not 'grow out of' their skin problem. In contrast, late-onset acne usually begins for the first time after the age of about twenty-five. Prior to this, there is usually no history of skin problems.

Both types of acne are thought to develop due to androgen hormones causing overstimulation of the oil glands.

Treatment strategies are broadly the same regardless of the age at which acne develops, although hormonal treatments vary between the sexes. So keep reading, as later in this chapter I'll give my advice on how best to tackle acne, no matter how old you are!

If acne is caused by hormone imbalance then shouldn't we check my hormone levels?

For most people, the answer to this question is 'no'.

The vast majority of adult women with acne have normal androgen levels on blood testing. The possible explanation for this is that levels are higher locally in the skin than in the bloodstream. There is scientific data that seems to be consistent with this which shows high levels of androgens around the sebaceous glands in skin. At this present time, there is no commercially available test to measure hormone levels around the oil gland and performing blood tests will add very little extra information as they are likely to be normal.

Are there any circumstances where a blood test is useful for acne?

Yes. Acne can sometimes occur as part of another medical problem and in these situations a blood test may be helpful. One such situation is when a condition known as polycystic ovarian syndrome (PCOS) is suspected.

PCOS is common and affects the way a woman's ovaries work. It is characterized by irregular periods, excess circulating androgens in the blood stream and ovaries that contain multiple fluid-filled sacs, or 'cysts'. Excess androgen can often lead to acne, oily skin and increased hair growth on the body but hair loss or thinning from the scalp. There are a number of other associations with the condition including weight gain and difficulties in trying to conceive. Not everyone suffers with every aspect of the condition and some people may only be troubled with stubborn acne. It is more common in certain ethnic groups, such as women from Asian communities.

If I suspect PCOS after speaking to, or examining, a patient in clinic then I will screen for the condition with hormonal blood tests and arrange an ultrasound scan to assess the ovaries. If you are concerned that you may have this condition, it might also be worthwhile having a chat with your GP as they too will be able to help you arrange these tests.

Why is my acne worse during my period?

This is a very common issue for women and one that many have simply come to accept as part and parcel of that time of the month. About two-thirds of acne-prone women will note worsening of their acne typically occurring anywhere from a week to a few days before the start of their period.

Though women have female hormones circulating through their bodies throughout their menstrual cycle (oestrogen predominating in the first half of the month and progesterone in the second half), the androgen testosterone is also present – albeit in smaller quantities – at all times. Shortly before the onset of menstrual bleeding, female hormones reach their lowest levels; the level of testosterone, however, remains fairly constant at all times and so is proportionally higher at this point. Such higher proportions of testosterone, in turn, are known to cause the changes in the skin's complexion that bring about acne. Unfortunately, us ladies are at the mercy of our hormonal cycles and there's not much we can do about them, even if we can treat the resultant acne.

I've heard that acne on my lower face is due to hormones. Is this true?

Fundamentally, all acne is hormonal, but in adult women it has often been reported – anecdotally – that it occurs more commonly on the lower half of the face, jawline, chin and neck. Actually, this is something I have noted from personal experience in my clinics; however, the scientific evidence is inconclusive on this point as we haven't yet determined the precise causes of such distribution.

On a similar note, some observations have suggested that acne type also varies by age in women, with adults usually suffering from tender, inflammatory (cystic) spots. They also seem to have fewer numbers of blackheads or whiteheads compared to teenagers. Again, however, not all scientific studies have confirmed this observation.

Will I grow out of acne?

Acne is probably best regarded as a chronic problem. Whilst some individuals will grow out of their skin problems, for many others, acne can cause much distress and recur over the years. Female adults with acne or those with underlying PCOS may exhibit more recalcitrant disease and higher treatment failure or relapse rates despite the use of standard therapies.

Speaking from my own personal experience, having suffered from acne for over twenty-five years, I think much of the distress that it causes stems from the belief that you should have grown out of it by the time you reach a certain age. It can be incredibly frustrating when it's back yet again after a round of what you thought was a successful treatment, but the reality is that it is often a condition that requires control rather than one amenable to a permanent cure. Acne is much easier to come to terms with when we realize that our real goal should be to minimize its impacts so that we can get on with life. If it returns, worry not; there are ways we can deal with it, and we needn't let it hold us back.

Is acne related to my diet?

The acne and diet story is controversial and interesting in equal measures. Before the 1960s, dietary advice to acne sufferers was a standard part of care and dermatologists recommended avoidance of sugary foods, carbonated drinks, chocolate and fat.

The turning point in the acne and diet story was in the late 1960s and early 1970s after two pivotal scientific studies, which reported the two were not connected. Diet was long forgotten by dermatologists until the turn of the 21st century with new research and a thorough critical analysis of the old data.

Although the total number of studies carried out over the past forty years is relatively small, there appears to be a growing body of support for the idea that certain types of food may aggravate acne. Emerging data suggests that high glycaemic index diets may have a role to play in how acne develops. There is also limited evidence that some dairy (in particular skimmed milk) may also have some influence.

a) High GI Foods

Foods which have a high glycaemic index (e.g. sugar, sweets, pizza, soft drinks, fast food, white bread) are rapidly absorbed by the body, leading to spikes in blood sugar or glucose levels. Raised circulating blood glucose levels promote the release of the hormone insulin and insulin-like growth factor 1 (IGF-1). Both increase sebum production and act on the body to produce more androgen hormone. These factors promote the development of acne, so if you're after clear skin (and I'd wager you are if you're reading this!), then you might consider limiting your intake of these naughty treats.

b) Dairy

The link between dairy as a cause or aggravating factor for acne is much weaker. There are a number of proposed hypotheses surrounding how dairy products may worsen skin disease. It is possible that dairy acts by a similar mechanism to diets rich in carbohydrates by promoting insulin and IGF-1 production. There are also suggestions that milk from dairy cows either naturally contains growth hormones or is treated with growth hormones. These can, in turn, increase androgen levels, which drive oil glands to release more sebum. I don't think everyone with acne needs to cut dairy out of their diet (I certainly don't!), but if you are one of the small group that notices a clear connection between eating dairy and breaking out in spots, then there would be a case to reduce or eliminate it from your diet. This is easier than it sounds given the wide variety of cow's milk alternatives readily available in shops and supermarkets.

The Western diet has often been researched as a potential cause for acne. Traditionally, it had been observed that Canadian Inuits and Zulu populations did not have acne. However, acne prevalence increased among the first group after adopting a diet of processed foods, beef and dairy. Among the Zulu population, acne development was attributed to migration from rural areas into cities. In contrast, native populations in Papua New Guinea and Paraguay that followed a 'paleo-like' diet did not have acne.

The ideal 'anti-acne' diet – if there is such a thing – would be low in sugar and refined carbohydrates. Vegetables and fruit with low glycaemic index (bananas, blueberries, broccoli, mushrooms, etc.) and fish high in omega-3 fatty acids will help. If there is concern that acne is being driven by diet, then consider carefully noting down everything you eat each day in a food diary for at least twelve weeks.

The evidence at the current time suggests that in a select group of individuals, diet may have a role to play in the development of acne. However, the scientific data is limited and the quality of clinical trials needs improvement. Most dermatologists will now recommend that acne should not be treated with diet alone but it may have an adjunctive role in some people alongside tried and tested, validated treatments.

Are there any supplements you can take for acne?

It is not uncommon in this day and age for people to want to trial a supplement for their skin and there is data from small studies regarding more 'natural' therapies. I am not an advocate of making recommendations that are not robustly supported by science, and think there are better treatments than taking supplements, but these oral agents are readily available in health food shops and may have a role to play, so why not give them a try:

- Nicotinamide (vitamin B3) – 750mg once daily
- Omega-3 fatty acids
- Zinc – 200mg daily of zinc gluconate or 400–600mg daily of zinc sulphate
- Vitamin A – 300,000 IU daily for women; 400,000 IU for men

If you are planning a pregnancy, breastfeeding or taking other prescribed medication then do not take these supplements without speaking to your family doctor or dermatologist first.

What products should I use for acne?

How to look after your skin is explained in more detail in chapter 2, 'Regular Skincare', and chapter 3, 'Skincare Regimes'. Most of us will try to manage our spots with products available over the counter rather than go straight to a dermatologist. Using the right types of formulations and ingredients is key.

Firstly, stay away from using facial oils as well as cleansers and moisturizers with thick creamy textures. Stick to light or gel-like formulations. Ideally the product should be labelled as 'non-comedogenic'; whilst this is not a guarantee the product will not make you break out, it is better than a product that is not labelled at all! Look for ingredients such as:

- salicylic acid
- glycolic acid
- zinc
- tea tree oil
- benzoyl peroxide
- niacinamide
- lactobionic acid
- retinol
- retinyl palmitate

If these products fail to control acne after a few weeks of use, it is time to seek advice from either your family doctor or dermatologist.

What are the treatments for acne?

There are a number of treatments available for acne depending on the severity and type of spots. Treatments can largely be broken down into creams and gels, tablets, and light-based devices.

a) Creams and gels

Retinoids: These are vitamin A-based products that stop skin cells from becoming sticky, reduce the blockage of pores and prevent blackheads from forming. When you first use these treatments, it is very common for skin irritation and redness to occur, so I usually recommend that treatment needs to be built up gradually. Start with a couple of applications a week initially, before building up to daily usage. Retinoids should be applied at night to clean skin. Sun protection should be worn in the day as the creams can cause sensitivity to sunlight. Some recommended products for purchase include NeoStrata Skin Active Retinol + NAG Complex, The Ordinary Retinol 1% and Medik8 Retinol 10 TR Serum.

Benzoyl peroxide: Benzoyl peroxide is a bactericidal agent that has the ability to reduce the amount of *P. acnes* bacteria in the skin. It is useful for both inflammatory and non-inflammatory acne spots. Products containing benzoyl peroxide can be obtained on prescription (e.g. Duac Gel or Epiduo Gel) or bought over the counter (e.g. Acnecide 5% Gel). These are used once or twice daily. A word of caution: it can cause irritation and bleach fabrics and hair.

Antibiotic creams and gels: These are often used for their antibacterial activity against *P. acnes*. Due to concerns about bacterial resistance they are not used alone and are usually combined with either retinoids or benzoyl peroxide. Antibiotic usage should, if possible, be limited to no more than twelve weeks.

Azelaic acid: This is not a standard treatment but it can be helpful in those that do not tolerate the other creams and gels. Azelaic acid would need to be prescribed by a dermatologist or GP if of a high concentration; lower concentrations can be bought over the counter.

b) Oral medications

If creams and gels fail to bring spots under control, then the next step is usually tablet treatment prescribed by a dermatologist or GP.

Antibiotic tablets: These have anti-inflammatory properties and activity against *P. acnes*. Oral antibiotics are usually used in combination with topical creams. Commonly used antibiotics in the

UK for acne include tetracycline, oxytetracycline, doxycycline and lymecycline. There is good evidence that these agents can reduce acne. Other antibiotics used include erythromycin, azithromycin and trimethoprim. Average treatment time is about twelve weeks. Increasingly, there is concern about bacterial resistance and effects on the gut microbiome so antibiotics should not be used indefinitely.

Hormonal therapies: The combined oral contraceptive pill ('the pill') can be used to control acne in women requiring contraception. Oestrogen in the contraceptive pill reduces sebum and androgen production. Data suggests that it can take up to three months to see skin benefits from the contraceptive pill. Certain pills are seen as more 'skin-friendly' and these include Yasmin and Dianette.

Spironolactone is another drug that can be used by specialists to treat acne in females. Its use in acne is 'off-label' which means the drug was licensed for another condition. Spironolactone has a useful role in female adults and those with PCOS. It should only be prescribed by a specialist with extensive experience of its use.

Isotretinoin (Roaccutane): Isotretinoin is a vitamin A-based drug that is highly effective in severe, recalcitrant acne with signs of scarring. It also has a role in acne that is resistant to treatment with other agents, relapses quickly after completion of antibiotic therapy or is having a profound psychological impact. In the UK, it can only be prescribed under the supervision of a dermatologist. Common side effects include dry lips, muscle soreness, sensitivity to sunlight and headaches. It is mandatory to have monitoring blood tests whilst taking the medication and female patients of child-bearing age are likely to need contraception as the drug is teratogenic. This means it will damage an unborn baby.

There was previously a question mark around the medication causing problems with depression and other mood problems but the most recent data suggests there is no link.

The difficulty with acne is that it is well known to cause problems with mood and self-esteem. It can be quite hard to tease out whether it is the acne itself (which must be severe by definition to qualify for isotretinoin) that is causing low mood or the initiation of the drug. For most, if anything, mood tends to improve with treatment – people feel better as their skin gets better. The majority of people tolerate the medication well and most side effects can be managed with the correct skincare or simply by reducing the dose.

Isotretinoin has received bad press in the past which is a real shame as the drug is safe and effective in expert hands and many people that would benefit from it have been poorly advised that the drug is dangerous.

c) Light and laser treatments

There is growing interest in new non-invasive therapies for acne. Light and laser therapies (photodynamic therapy, blue light, intense pulsed light) are commercially available and the results are encouraging. The treatments can be expensive as a course of treatment and maintenance is often required, and it is also possible for acne to come back once the treatment is stopped. However, there is no doubt that these have a place for those that do not, or cannot, take oral medications. These treatments appear promising, but further studies are undoubtedly needed to assess their value.

The beauty industry, however, remains a step ahead and there are already a number of home acne light devices available commercially, many of which are very affordable. These include the Neutrogena Light Therapy Acne Mask and the Lumie Clear Acne Treatment Light, both of which I have purchased and used alongside other treatments. My feeling is that they may have a role for those with mild acne or as a holding measure for those awaiting a dermatology appointment. They are not, however, a miracle cure and the treatments do need to be repeated regularly to be effective; therefore, be aware that you'll need to set aside time for their use in your daily routine as per the manufacturer's guidance.

I've suddenly developed a huge spot two days before my wedding. What can I do?

It is bad enough on a normal day to wake up to an angry volcano on your face, but just before an important social event can be soul-destroying, and this is only magnified a hundredfold when you're going to be the centre of attention. I still can't bear to look at my graduation photos thanks to the unsightly beast standing proud on my forehead.

But panic not! The good news (and if only I'd known this when I graduated!) is that there is a treatment for this. Dermatologists can inject acne cysts with a small amount of steroid or cortisone. This feels a bit uncomfortable but the spot goes down very quickly in a matter of forty-eight hours. It needs to be done by an experienced dermatologist as there are risks of an indented scar, pigmentation change and prominent blood vessels appearing, but it is good as a quick fix just before your big day.

I think it is also worth making the point that if you are getting a lot of spots, this is not the best solution as you probably do need a longer-term approach. If you have any concerns, make sure you see a dermatologist a few months before the wedding to give them enough time to sort it out for you.

I'm thinking about getting pregnant. What should I do about my acne?

Many of my patients are in their early to mid-thirties and suffering with troublesome cystic acne. It is quite clear to me within minutes of seeing them that acne is literally ruining their lives. The acne makes them feel unattractive and their confidence and self-esteem suffer as a result. They already know deep down that they need medication as they have exhausted all of the skincare and diet options long before booking their appointment with me.

Yet many are at an age where having children is also on their radar. I see many women in serious relationships, about to get engaged or married, and thinking about starting a family. If conception is on the cards, it immediately puts many effective acne medications off-limits.

A common theme that emerges when I probe further is that many women feel ashamed to say out loud that they want to get their skin sorted before becoming pregnant. There can still be societal expectations that women of a certain age should prioritize having children, and they can fear being judged by a significant other, family or friends. Many will ask me directly, 'Do you think it's shallow that I would delay having a baby because I want to get my acne treated first?'

I think this question reflects the fact that society still thinks of acne as just a cosmetic concern. This is wrong; it is not. Acne can have a number of detrimental impacts on mental health, and these must not be underestimated.

Suppose you are trying for a baby, get pregnant and then opt to breastfeed whilst having cystic acne – that could potentially mean two years (maybe more) where you would be unable to have effective tablet options to treat your skin. Based on how your skin makes you feel right now, are you prepared to wait that long for effective treatment?

I find this question difficult to ask and I'm fully aware it's also very difficult to answer. I cannot – and should not – make your decisions for you, but I can give you the options and my honest, expert advice.

Everyone deserves good mental health, and the chance to lead a happy and fulfilling life, whether a prospective mother or not. Mood and self-esteem can impact your existing relationships, but for new parents it also affects the environment in which your baby will grow up. From a more practical perspective, the longer cystic acne is left untreated, the more likely you are to develop scarring. Acne scarring is significantly harder – and significantly more expensive – to treat than the acne itself.

As is often the way with life, there is no easy – or correct – solution to this. I have had a number of patients tell me they are at breaking point with their acne. I actively encourage these patients to go away and speak to their partners and close ones to see if delaying a pregnancy by six to nine months is acceptable for them. For some it is, and they treat their acne first; their mood and psycho-logical well-being improves as their skin gets better. They find they are then in a happier and healthier place for having children. For others, this is not so. They make the decision that having a baby comes first and the acne comes afterwards. This is fine too. Ultimately, you must do what's right for you and your loved ones, and resist being coerced in either direction.

I'm pregnant. What acne treatments can I safely use?

This is a tough one. There is very little that is licensed for acne in pregnancy. The oral antibiotic erythromycin com-bined with the prescription cream azelaic acid are both safe to use. Stick to skincare products that contain glycolic acid but avoid salicylic acid-based products (which could theoretically contribute to birth defects). Non-medicinal approaches such as chemical peels and lasers may also be an option that some experts may offer.

Why do I get acne on my back?

'Bacne', as it is popularly known, causes problems for both sexes and can lead to much embarrassment when it comes to swimming, getting undressed in communal changing rooms or when in front of a partner.

It is surprisingly common and has a tendency to affect men more than women. About half of people that suffer with acne will find that their back is also affected. It is unusual, but not impossible, to get back acne in the absence of facial acne. As the skin of the back is particularly thick, it is a site prone to developing deep, red, painful spots.

Back acne is caused in the same way as normal acne: hormones and genetics. However, it can also occur due to frequent gym sessions where increased heat, sweat and synthetic clothing result in occlusion of the skin. Make sure you shower as soon as possible after exercise and definitely do not hang around in sweaty gym clothes any longer than you have to! If you are still breaking out, get medical help as the treatments for back acne are otherwise the same as for facial acne.

Why do I get spots on my bum?

They're not often talked about, but spots on the buttocks are surprisingly common. Whilst they can look like acne, they are usually caused by another skin problem known as folliculitis. Hair follicles can become blocked, inflamed and infected, leading to a spotty rash that can be itchy at times. The trend for 'athleisure' does not help, and sitting around in tight, synthetic, occlusive clothing can be a cause for some. Gym kit should ideally be left for the gym and not regular daywear!

How do I get rid of my blackheads?

Blackheads are often incorrectly thought to be pores blocked with dirt, which gives them their black appearance. In actual fact, skin oil contains a pigment known as melanin within it. As the oil blocks the pore on the skin surface, melanin oxidizes with air and turns black, hence the black appearance and the name 'blackhead'.

a) Home treatments

Retinoid creams and gels can be helpful in reducing blackheads. These need to be used for eight to twelve weeks before real benefit is apparent, so definitely aren't a quick fix. They are available over the counter and on prescription (e.g. Differin).

It can be helpful to exfoliate the skin on a weekly basis to remove the upper layer of dead skin cells and reduce the formation of blackheads. I wouldn't recommend doing this more than once per week as you may irritate the skin and make it worse.

b) Clinic-based treatments

Steam extractions can also be of benefit. Steam is used to loosen the blockage within the pores and then an extractor tool can be used to remove black-heads. This can be carried out by a trained facialist or aesthetician. Its benefits are that it can reduce the number of future inflamed acne spots and immediately creates a sense of 'decongestion' or unblocking of the skin. However, it carries a risk of damage to the skin and can make deep-seated spots worse. It really, therefore, needs to be done by a trained professional rather than by yourself, having learned the technique from a YouTube video. In either case, as blackheads re-form over time, the procedure will need to be repeated.

Chemical peels can also be used for blackheads with good results and there are many types of superficial peels available (e.g. glycolic acid and salicylic acid). These chemicals are applied to the surface of the skin and cause an accelerated type of exfoliation. Again, it is important to see a trained professional as not all peels are suitable for all skin types and certain types of acne may not respond.

Blackheads can also be combatted with a heat treatment known as electrodesiccation in a dermatology practice. A fine metal electrode heats up the skin and removes the blackheads. This treatment is sometimes used by dermatologists to reduce blackheads before starting their patient on stronger acne medication such as isotretinoin (Roaccutane).

My spots get better in the sun. Do I need to use sunscreen?

In the 1950s, sun and sun lamps were used to treat acne. I see many patients who have had this treatment in the past as they have since developed skin cancer from the ultraviolet light exposure.

Many people feel their acne improves in sunlight and there are a number of reasons for this. Firstly, as your skin tans, the redness of the acne becomes relatively less visible. Secondly, ultraviolet light from the sun suppresses inflammation in the skin, which can drive acne. The problem is that suppression of the skin's normal immune response can leave you more vulnerable to developing skin cancers further down the line.

So the answer is a resounding yes; you do need to wear sunscreen. Many people feel that greasy sunscreens can actually make their acne worse and it is important to ensure your dermatologist recommends products that are designed specifically for acne-prone skin. My personal favourites are Heliocare 360 Gel Oil-free SPF 50, Avène Cleanance Solaire SPF 30 and Skinceuticals Mineral Matte UV Defense SPF 30. As with regular skincare, avoid thick creams and opt for gels and oil-free formulations. Some people find that mineral sunscreens containing zinc or titanium work best for their skin.

When should I seek help for acne?

There is no simple answer to this, but no one should be suffering in silence because of their skin. If you have tried over-the-counter products that have failed to work, your acne is affecting how you feel or is causing scarring or pigmentation, then these are all signs that you should be seeking medical attention.

The operative term here is 'medical attention'; I frequently see distraught patients who have spent hundreds to thousands of pounds on their skin concerns because they have not received proper guidance from a qualified professional. In a recent clinic I saw a patient in her late twenties who heart-breakingly confessed to having parted with £4,000 – money she could not comfortably afford to spend – on skincare products and bogus treatments that did nothing at all. When I explained why these had not worked, and then outlined how I could help, she was so over-whelmed by the realization that she would not have to live with her acne for ever that she burst into tears. She is one of my many patients who have a similar tale to tell, and it infu-riates me no end that there are individuals out there who will take advantage of others' skin misery for financial gain.

What are the psychological effects associated with acne?

Acne has been linked to a large number of mood problems and these should not be underestimated. If you are suffering, or know someone else that is, it is important to encourage them to receive help. Acne can cause problems with self-esteem and body image, it can lead to social withdrawal and difficulty in forming relationships, and also cause avoidance behaviour, embarrassment and depression.

A survey in 2015 commissioned by the British Skin Foundation, the UK's largest skin charity, of over 2,000 acne sufferers revealed that nearly 20 per cent had thought about or considered suicide as a result of their acne. A whopping 40 per cent reported bullying as a result of their skin condition. These findings are not to be taken lightly.

ACNE SCARRING

My first experience with a dermatologist to address acne was at the age of fourteen. My face at this stage had at least twenty to thirty deep spots at any one time. I remember, as I used to count them. I recall sitting in front of a mirror and trying to cover the spots with my fingertips – mainly trying to imagine what I might look like without them – and then very quickly running out of fingers.

The consultant dermatologist was old and male. In retrospect, I was young and I don't think he was anywhere near as old as I thought he was. I was distressed not only by my acne but also the deep, angry pits on both sides of my cheeks. He barely addressed me during most of the consultation and spoke directly with my mother. Before we were ushered out, I plucked up the courage to ask him one question: 'Will the scars get better?' He finally turned to look at me and gave me a one-word answer.

'No.'

I think I burst into tears at that stage. But that was it; the conversation was over. I realize now, in my older age, doing exactly the same job as he did, he had no idea how to handle a teenage girl or the effect his manner had on my confidence. More to the point, he was wrong.

Once acne scarring develops, it can be difficult to treat and the skin may never look entirely the same way as before *but* there are a number of good treatments, often used in combination, that can absolutely help the skin.

Who gets acne scarring?

Acne scarring affects about 20 per cent of people with acne. It can be more difficult to treat than the acne itself, and it is more likely to occur with deep acne lesions and if you pick or squeeze spots.

Why does scarring occur?

Acne scarring typically occurs as a result of spots that cause deep inflammation (nodules and cysts). Inflammation and its resolution can result in a number of skin surface abnormalities:

- Deposition of new collagen causing uneven surface elevation of the skin.
- Tethering of the skin surface resulting in small depressions or 'pits'.

- Permanently enlarged or dilated blood vessels as part of the body's natural wound-healing response to inflammation, resulting in redness.
- Damage to skin cells which causes the release of the pigment melanin, which in turn causes a brown discolouration.

The altered skin texture and colour contrasts sharply with normal surrounding 'unscarred' skin and therefore easily attracts the eye's attention.

Types of acne scar

Scars can either be raised (elevated) or indented (depressed) from the skin surface.

a) Elevated scars

There are two types of raised scars: hypertrophic and keloid. Both types occur due to the overgrowth of dense fibrous tissue after healing of a skin injury. Generally speaking, hypertrophic scars are the same size as the spot that caused them, but keloid scars extend beyond the limits of the acne lesion. Keloid scarring is more common in skin of colour and typically occurs on the shoulders, angle of the jaw and chest area. It usually requires medical intervention to soften or flatten the areas.

b) Depressed scars

There are three main types of depressed, or 'atrophic', acne scarring.

Ice pick scars: These are deep, narrow, pitted scars usually less than 2mm wide at their base.

Boxcar scars: These are broad depressions with sharply defined edges. The scars can be several millimetres wide and can result in a 'crateriform' appearance of the skin.

Rolling scars: These are broad depressions with sloping edges, which leave the skin with an undulating appearance.

Acne of the forehead and mid to upper cheeks typically results in multiple small ice pick scars. Acne of thicker areas of skin, such as the lower cheeks, chin and jawline, usually results in larger and deeper scars. Many individuals suffering from acne scarring are likely to have a combination of the different subtypes.

How can acne scarring be treated?

Whilst some acne scarring will improve over time, the skin contour does not usually completely normalize. There are a number of methods that can be used to treat acne scarring if it is causing distress. Typically, a combination of treatments is required to get the best result. This can be due to an individual having multiple types of scars on their skin simultaneously, but it should also be stressed that specific treatments, though they contribute to the improvement of the scar type to a degree, can only go so far when used in isolation.

For the best results, therefore, a sufferer needs access to the full suite of available treatments, together with an expert cosmetic dermatologist who can both select the right combination and administer them effectively and safely. Effective scar treatments will not come cheaply, and I would really stress the point that prevention is much better – and much less expensive – than cure in this instance. So get the acne treated as soon as possible before scarring has a chance to get a foothold. If, unfortunately, this is not an option as you already have indented scars, I would wholeheartedly recommend against throwing your money at creams, lotions, potions and popular oils as – despite what the packaging may claim – they simply will not be effective against such scarring. Skincare in this context would be a false economy; your money would be better spent getting expert opinion from a dermatologist or plastic surgeon.

a) Steroid injections

Steroid injections are often used to flatten raised scars so are ideal for the hypertrophic and keloid varieties. Small injections, usually with the agent triamcinolone, are placed directly into the scar. Depending on the size of the scar, several treatment sessions may be required and these are usually done a few weeks apart. This is a safe procedure but should only be carried out by an expert due to various risks including skin thinning and pigmentation change.

b) Chemical peels

Chemical peels, which are discussed in more detail in chapter 7, 'Anti-ageing Treatments', can also be effective for treating minor scarring. This is particularly true if medium to deep peels are used. Chemical peels use an acidic solution to damage the affected layers of skin. Redness, peeling and tightness of the skin occurs with deeper peels, and after several treatments minor scarring can be improved as new, healthy skin is revealed.

c) Surgical treatments

Surgical treatments, such as subcision and punch excision, can be useful methods for treating indented acne scars. Ice pick and boxcar scars can be removed by punch excision. This method uses a tool known as a punch biopsy to cut out the scarred area under local anaesthetic, with the resulting wound closed by a small suture or stitch. Round, irregular scars can be turned into flat slit-like scars with this technique.

d) Subcision

This will treat rolling scars. A needle is inserted into the skin after appropriate numbing and used to break up the fibrous bands that are causing tethering of the skin. This causes release of the depressed scar.

e) Dermabrasion

Dermabrasion is a skin resurfacing technique that surgically abrades the upper layers of skin, often by the use of a rotating tool. This triggers a wound-healing response in the affected layers and can be useful for smoothing out very superficial scarring.

f) Microneedling

Medical microneedling is a clinic-based treatment also sometimes known as collagen induction therapy. The skin is numbed using local anaesthetic cream and a device is used to make multiple small pin-point injuries to the skin which heal within two days. Micro-injury to the skin is thought to promote new collagen production and may have a role in treating minor depressed acne scarring. Usually, multiple treatments about four to six weeks apart are required.

g) Dermal fillers

Dermal fillers are products injected under the skin surface, mainly for their anti-ageing effects; again, these are discussed in more detail in chapter 7, 'Anti-ageing Treatments'. The most commonly used fillers contain hyaluronic acid, a naturally occurring sugar found in the body that provides hydration and plumping of the skin. Synthetic hyaluronic dermal fillers can be effective treatment for rolling acne scars. These are injected into the skin and, depending on the type of product used, can temporarily lift the scar for six months or so. This treatment is often combined with subcision and not suitable for ice pick scars. There is a risk of bruising, swelling, discomfort and bumps. Agents other than hyaluronic acid can be used in experienced hands, such as fillers containing calcium hydroxylapatite.

h) Trichloroacetic Acid Chemical Reconstruction of Skin Scars (TCA CROSS)

This is another clinic procedure that can be useful for treating depressed acne scars. Small amounts of trichloroacetic acid (TCA) are deposited directly into the scars in high concentration (70–100 per cent). A local inflammatory reaction is triggered, resulting in new collagen production into the scarred area. It can have a useful role in treating ice pick, boxcar and rolling scars. The procedure is usually well-tolerated by patients with little complication if performed by an expert. Often, multiple sessions may be required.

i) Laser therapies

Now this is something I have personal experience of. The florid cystic acne I had as a teenager left extensive scarring on both my cheeks. I didn't treat this for many years, as the spots continued intermittently over the years and my preconceptions about the cost and the downtime put me off until a few years ago when I visited Canada to further my laser training. Whilst I was out there, I ended up having the procedure done myself (and am honestly kicking myself for not having had it sooner!). I found the treatment effective, with tolerable discomfort, and my skin was red and peeling for several days afterwards. However, over the following months, there was a visible improvement. There is still some minor scarring left behind, although this doesn't bother me so I've opted not to have further sessions at this stage (though I may change my mind in the future!).

There are multiple laser therapies available that can improve acne scarring. The best laser device for a given patient depends on their skin type and the nature and extent of the scarring.

Laser resurfacing for depressed facial scars can be carried out by ablative lasers such as Erbium:YAG (don't let the name worry you!) and carbon dioxide lasers. Ablative lasers have a two-fold action: they destroy the upper layer of skin (epidermis) and use heat to damage the deeper layers (dermis). A wound-healing response is prompted in the skin.

Before the treatment, an anaesthetic cream is normally applied for thirty to sixty minutes to numb the area. After the treatment and in the following days, the skin is likely to be red, raw and swollen and will require regular moisturizing with heavy ointments. Healing can take seven to ten days depending on the type and depth of laser used. Lasers may not be the treatment of choice in ethnic skin due to the risk of pigmentation problems after the procedure; caution and an experienced practitioner is therefore needed.

Over the years, non-ablative laser devices have gained popularity. Whilst they are not as effective as ablative lasers, they have an excellent safety profile and quicker recovery time. Non-ablative lasers do not affect the epidermis, but use heat to promote new collagen production in the dermis.

Modern-day ablative lasers are often 'fraction-ated'. This means they deliver heat into the skin through numerous tiny, deep columns known as microthermal treatment zones, with areas of normal, untreated skin between them. The skin heals more quickly with this fractionation than if the entire area was treated and the complication rate is also much lower. Often, a series of treatments is necessary. There are a number of non-ablative fractionated lasers used for acne scarring. These have complicated names (and I won't bore you with technical details), but common ones to look out for include Erbium:glass 1540nm, 1064 Q-switched (QS) Nd:YAG, 1450 nm diode and 1320 Nd:YAG.

Who should not have acne scarring treatment?

If there is any evidence of active acne then scarring treatment should not be carried out. If acne is ongoing then scars are going to continue to develop despite scar treatment. This is therefore a waste of time and money as the sufferer ends up chasing their tail trying to get rid of existing scars as new ones continually develop. Also, many scarring treatments can cause a flare-up of pre-existing acne.

Treating the skin should be thought of as a two-step process in this scenario. The acne needs to be switched off first before one embarks on scar treatments.

Choosing the right person to do scar treatments

For acne scarring (and, indeed, any scar treatment), it is important to choose a practitioner listed as a dermatologist or plastic surgeon on the General Medical Council specialist register. The best practitioner to perform acne scarring treatments is likely to be a cosmetic dermatologist. If there is active acne, then a dermatologist is also the only person that is strictly able to provide you with all prescription medications before scar treatments take place.

When choosing a cosmetic dermatologist, it is worthwhile making sure he or she has access to most or all of the treatment options discussed. Realistically, it is often the case that combination treatments are required to produce best results; access to lasers is therefore important. Before signing up to any treatment, your dermatologist should be able to give you the pros, cons and alternatives. It can sometimes be a false economy signing up for multiple sessions of cheaper, less invasive treatments than a single session of something which, at first glance, seems expensive.

Post-inflammatory change

I often have patients come to clinic concerned about brown or red marks on their skin after acne. However, when you feel the skin, the surface is flat; there are no raised or indented areas of scarring. These marks are very common following acne and although often mistaken for scars they are not in fact representative of true scarring. They occur due to inflammation and often look red in paler skins (post-inflammatory erythema) and dark brown in pigmented skin (post-inflammatory hyperpigmentation).

Post-inflammatory change will usually fade over a period of months with no treatment. Over-the-counter creams and gels containing niacinamide, glycolic acid, kojic acid, arbutinin, vitamin C, azelaic acid and retinoids can speed this process up. Contrary to popular belief, these treatments and other popular face oils will not help scarring that is indented where skin damage is too deep. Provided the acne has stopped, red and brown marks can also be treated effectively in clinic with microneedling, peels and laser.

PORES

Many of us have an obsession with pore size. Magnifying mirrors don't help and it is easy to become fixated on those troublesome little holes, particularly if you're a woman from the oily skin gang. There are many misconceptions about what pores are, what they do and how we can supposedly shrink them. Whilst not a dangerous skin issue, pores cause a great deal of cosmetic concern and I see many women approaching me for treatment.

So, let's start with what they really are. Pores are a natural part of the skin structure and where oil glands and hair follicles open on to the skin surface. The biggest myth I hear about pores is that you can change their size. I have lost count of how many times on Instagram I see cosmetic doctors, bloggers and glossy magazines mistakenly reporting that a product or treatment opens pores or shrinks pores. Pores do not have muscles around their outside that can contract or relax to change their size.

Pores are more visible in those with oily skin and acne. In women, hormonal factors may have a part to play and there are studies which show that pores become more prominent during ovulation, possibly due to a surge in the hormone progesterone. Pores can also appear for the first time with advancing age. Ultraviolet radiation and other environmental factors like pollution damage collagen in the skin over time. Loss of the skin's structural support around the pore can make it more noticeable than before. Pore prominence seems to vary across ethnic groups, with Chinese women coming out most favourably.

Whilst actual pore size itself can't be changed, there are a number of methods to help reduce the appearance of size. The scientific evidence is limited and few people have carried out large clinical trials, but there are a number of methods commonly used by cosmetic dermatologists that can make pores less visible.

a) Retinoid cream

Retinoid creams have a great many benefits, which is why I mention them in several sections of this book for their effectiveness in preventing blackheads, fading pigmentation and promoting the growth of new collagen. Prescription retinoids such as tretinoin 0.05 per cent can also improve the appearance of pores. They really are the miracle skincare agent.

Retinoids can cause dryness and irritation and their use should be built up gradually. If you do not tolerate a prescription-strength retinoid then an over-the-counter retinol (e.g. 0.5 per cent or 1 per cent) is worth a trial. It is weaker but will cause fewer problems with skin sensitivity.

b) Chemical peels

Glycolic acid peels at strengths of 35–40 per cent done at regular intervals can help the appearance of pores. Peels at this strength need to be carried out in a medical or clinical setting. Most over-the-counter glycolic acid preparations come in significantly lower concentrations.

c) Oral medications

Anecdotal and observational data suggests that certain oral medications can help with pore appearance by regulating oil production. These include medications that act on reducing androgens (male hormones) or low doses of oral retinoid drugs. These should only be taken if prescribed under the guidance of a consultant dermatologist.

d) Lasers, radio-frequency and ultrasound devices

These devices deliver heat or ultrasound energy to the deeper skin layers in a controlled fashion. This generates new collagen production and improves skin elasticity to reduce the appearance of pore size.

Whilst a number of options exist, the simplest method is to start with topical creams or seek advice from a cosmetic dermatologist who has access to, and experience in, a number of treatment methods.

ROSACEA

The name rosacea comes to us from the Latin *rosaceus*, meaning 'rose-coloured', and is so called because one of its most distinctive visual symptoms is a redness of the nose and cheeks. Rosacea is probably the second commonest skin concern that patients visit me to address, but is a funny one in so far as many sufferers are not aware that it is a recognized medical condition. Rather, they assume their skin merely happens to be more red (and sensitive) than others'.

Let's look at rosacea in a bit of detail.

What is rosacea?

Rosacea is a common inflammatory skin condition that affects the face. It is characterized by redness which usually comes and goes, but it can over time become permanent. Other characteristic features include frequent blushing or flushing, spots that can look like acne and enlarged, visible blood vessels. Those who suffer also report problems with sensitive skin. Less often, it is possible to develop thickening of skin, usually of the nose. Not everyone will have issues with each one of these signs and symptoms and the severity can be variable. It usually worsens with time if left untreated.

Rosacea was previously and incorrectly known as 'acne rosacea'. This term is no longer used, as it is not related to acne. There is no blood or skin test for rosacea, and diagnosis is usually made based on its appearance.

Who gets rosacea?

The typical rosacea sufferer is female, aged thirty to sixty, with fair skin type or Celtic origin. It is more common in women than men but when men are affected by the condition, it can be far more severe. Men are more likely to have problems with skin thickening, particularly of the nose (rhinophyma). Rosacea can affect darker skin types but this is seen less frequently. It can be difficult to appreciate the severity of redness in ethnic skin types: redness does not show up as much on dark skin compared to white skin.

What is the cause of rosacea?

Rosacea remains poorly understood. We still do not know the exact cause, although there are several hypothesized factors, including hyper-reactive blood vessels that dilate more easily than they should. Other possibilities include an abnormal immune response in the skin, the presence of microscopic skin mites known as Demodex, genetics and the presence of inflammatory factors. The likelihood is that all of these have a role to play in causation.

Does rosacea affect anywhere other than the face?

Rosacea is predominantly a condition of the central face: the nose, cheeks and chin. In some sufferers, it can also affect the eyes, and is known as 'ocular rosacea'. It can result in the eyes becoming watery, red and irritated. The skin of the eyelids can become swollen and styes are common.

Ongoing medical research into rosacea suggests it may also be related to other medical conditions associated with inflammation. It has also been linked to migraines and gastro-oesophageal reflux, which can cause heartburn. Those who suffer with severe rosacea may be at a higher risk of heart disease.

Is there a cure for rosacea?

Unfortunately, rosacea is a chronic disease so there is no cure. It goes through cycles of remission (where it can get better) and flare (where it can get worse). Over time, it is possible to get worsening of the condition if no treatment is given. That said, it can be kept under control using a variety of methods.

What makes rosacea worse?

There are several well-recognized triggers for rosacea that can make it worse. The biggest culprit is sun exposure, which can affect the skin in over 80 per cent of those who suffer. Other common triggers include emotional stress, change or extremes of temperature, wind, exercise, alcohol, cheese, spicy food, hot drinks and certain skincare products (detailed below).

How is rosacea treated?

One of the most crucial aspects of managing rosacea is adequate sun protection. Daily sunscreen with a minimum SPF of 30 offering protection against UVA and UVB rays from the sun is vital. Sun exposure can drive the condition and this vital step must be incorporated into daily routine.

UV rays have the ability to penetrate cloud cover so sunscreen should be worn in the winter months too.

There are also a number of prescription agents and other forms of treatment that can be used to control rosacea.

a) Creams and gels

There are several cream therapies for rosacea. These can reduce inflammatory bumps or spots, reduce redness, improve skin sensitivity and reduce the number and intensity of flare-ups. These include agents such as:

- azelaic acid
- ivermectin
- brimonidine
- metronidazole

b) Oral medications

Inflammatory rosacea that consists of many red bumps (papules and pustules) responds well to oral antibiotics. These are used for three to four months or until remission is achieved. Standard antibiotics include tetracyclines and erythromycin. These particular drugs have been used for decades and have a good safety profile. Antibiotics in the context of rosacea are used more for their anti-inflammatory, rather than their antibacterial, effects.

For severe cases of rosacea, the medication isotretinoin (Roaccutane) can be used to reduce bumps and inflammation. It is usually used in lower doses than for acne treatment and can produce good results. Careful monitoring under the guidance of an experienced dermatologist is required.

Flushing or blushing can cause extreme frustration for many and there are oral tablets that can help with this symptom. Medications such as clonidine and propranolol are usually given to control this challenging aspect of rosacea.

c) Laser and light treatments

These treatments can be highly effective for treating the redness and enlarged blood vessels (telangiectasia) associated with rosacea. Intense pulsed light (IPL) and pulsed-dye laser (PDL) are used most commonly. A course of treatment is required and this could range from three to six sessions carried out at monthly to six-weekly intervals. Redness often recurs over time and maintenance treatment (e.g. annually) may be required. The treatments are not particularly painful and can be carried out by an experienced cosmetic dermatologist with laser experience. The benefit of seeing a dermatologist is that he or she will also be able to provide other aspects of rosacea care, such as prescribing appropriate creams and oral treatments. Before arranging appointments, ensure that your treating dermatologist has access to light and laser devices.

Is there anything I should avoid?

Trigger avoidance is key in rosacea. Whilst this may not always be possible, limitation of triggers is the next best thing. Sun avoidance and adequate protection is of value to everyone but other triggers are likely to be specific to each individual.

Many people with rosacea can be sensitive to ingredients in skincare products. It's a good idea to trial a new product on a small area of skin first to make sure it does not cause redness, burning or irritation. Behind the ear, on the side of the neck or the hairless part of the forearms are a sensible place to do this.

It can be helpful to avoid skincare products that contain alcohol, witch hazel, menthol, camphor, fragrance, peppermint, eucalyptus, propylene glycol, parabens, sodium lauryl sulphate, glycolic and salicylic acid. Retinoid creams, which are often used for their anti-ageing properties, should be used with caution.

What type of sunscreen should I use?

I cannot emphasize this enough: broad-spectrum sunscreen with an SPF of 30 should be worn on a daily basis for those with rosacea, even in the winter months. As the product is being worn every day it needs to be non-irritating to the skin. Sunscreens containing dimethicone or cyclomethicone are often tolerated better than products without. Alternatively, many rosacea sufferers find that mineral or physical sunscreens suit them better than those containing chemicals. These products can easily be identified as they usually contain either titanium or zinc.

How should I look after my skin?

The skincare regime of someone with rosacea needs to be kept relatively simple. The more you manipulate the skin and layer products, the greater the opportunity for unnecessary irritation.

Skin should be cleansed morning and evening. The ideal cleanser leaves minimal residue on the skin, is 'non-comedogenic' and has a neutral or slightly acidic pH. In general, scrubs and toners should be avoided. If using a rinse-off cleanser, wash with cool or lukewarm water. Examples of suitable products include: Avène Extremely Gentle Cleanser, La Roche-Posay Toleriane Cleanser, Eucerin Redness Relief Soothing Cleanser and CeraVe Hydrating Cleanser.

Moisturizing daily in the morning, and evening if needed, is important to maintain skin softness and elasticity. Some people with rosacea may have naturally dry skin and others may be using prescription medications that can lead to dryness. Regular moisturizing (e.g. with La Roche-Posay Rosaliac Anti-Redness Moisturizer) will improve hydration and the skin's natural barrier function. Opt for creams rather than lotions.

What types of make-up can I use?

Individuals with rosacea should avoid the use of water-proof cosmetic products, as their removal often requires the use of solvents that can cause irritation. Mineral-based make-up, such as Dermablend Cover Crème Foundation or Colorescience, is useful as it often contains inert ingredients. Prominent redness can be camouflaged by using products that contain a green tint. Alternatively, a green-tinted primer can be applied to the skin before applying an oil-free foundation.

Can diet help?

Alcohol, cheese, spicy foods and hot drinks have been implicated in triggering rosacea, and limiting these can help with the skin. Both cayenne and red peppers, furthermore, can be potential triggers in addition to citrus fruits and tomatoes.

Dietary supplementation with omega-3 fatty acids and flaxseed oil seems to help ocular rosacea and may also have a role in reducing inflammation of the skin.

What are the psychological effects of rosacea?

Facial redness and bumps can have a huge impact on emotional wellness. The condition can be stigmatizing as many people incorrectly believe it is related to excess alcohol intake. Emotional stress can trigger flushing, which can be a source of great embarrassment to those that are suffering. Anxiety and depression have also been recognized in association with the condition.

A patient visited me in clinic who was concerned about her skin redness getting worse over the last twenty to thirty years. As it worsened, she had become increasingly self-conscious, even going so far as to change her job so that she worked from home full-time in order to avoid day-to-day contact with others. Throughout this considerable span of time, she had been completely unaware that she was suffering from rosacea or, indeed, that treatments existed. Starting her on the correct skincare, prescription treatments and laser was life-changing for her, but her story powerfully illustrates the psychological effects of skin conditions, and the dramatic impact they can have on everyday living.

When should I see a doctor?

Any skin condition that is limiting daily life or social interaction, or causing problems with mood or confidence, should be discussed with a GP or dermatologist. If the bumps, redness, flushing or skin sensitivity fail to improve with over-the-counter skincare products, it is a sign that it is worthwhile speaking to a doctor. If your GP offers you treatment and the skin does not improve after four to six weeks then consider seeking the opinion of a cosmetic dermatologist with access to IPL and laser technology.

PIGMENTATION

Pigmentation problems constitute one of the main reasons patients attend my dermatology clinics. They can cause great cosmetic concern and affect quality of life, particularly when society values smooth, unblemished skin as a sign of health and beauty. There are two main types of pigmentation problem: melasma and age spots (solar lentigines).

I recently saw a patient in her forties who had been troubled with dark patches on her forehead, cheeks and upper lip for seven years, starting during her last pregnancy. She was extremely self-conscious, particularly of the skin over her upper lip, feeling it looked like a moustache. She refused to go outdoors without heavy make-up and was reluctant to remove it, even at home in front of her husband and small children. A familiar story: she had spent a lot of money on over-the-counter cosmetic products promising to brighten the skin, but had seen no improvement. Her self-esteem was at an all-time low and she had finally decided to seek help. She was suffering from a condition called melasma, for which I subsequently treated her and helped improve her quality of life.

Melasma

Melasma is a chronic acquired skin disorder characterized by symmetrical, brown pigmentation that usually affects the face. The majority of cases are seen in women and can result in considerable social and emotional stress to the sufferer. It usually develops between the ages of twenty and forty, and is more common in olive tones or darker skin types. Affected areas typically include the forehead, cheeks and upper lip. There are a number of recognized triggers including sun exposure, pregnancy, hormonal treatments (combined oral contraceptive pill, intrauterine devices, implants, etc.), certain medications, and an underactive thyroid gland.

Melasma has a very typical appearance and does not require additional tests to make the diagnosis. Dense pigmentation deposits can lie in the epidermis (upper layer) or dermis (lower layer), but often both skin layers are affected. Dermatologists sometimes use a Wood lamp (a type of UV lamp) examination to try and determine in which layer the pigment lies. If melasma predominantly affects the upper layers of the skin, it is more likely to respond to cream treatments than if the melasma is deeper.

Melasma can be recurrent and refractory (stubborn or poorly responsive to treatment), which makes it difficult to address. For most people, treatments can produce reasonable to good results but the condition is likely to come back over time. Sadly, there is no definitive cure.

Melasma treatments

a) Creams and gels

Hydroquinone: Prescription agents containing hydroquinone 2–5 per cent remain a standard therapy for treating melasma. It works by blocking the chemical pathway that produces melanin (pigment). Hydroquinone cream is applied at night to affected areas for three to four months. Dermatologists usually use hydroquinone in combination with retinoid agents (tretinoin) to improve penetration and a mild topical steroid to reduce irritation. About 25 per cent of those that use this mixture will experience burning and irritation of the skin. This is not a reason to stop treatment altogether, but use would need to be gradually built up as tolerated. Hydroquinone-based products should not be used for prolonged periods of time as there is a risk of developing ochronosis, a permanent bluish/grey pigmentation of the skin.

Hydroquinone is generally considered to be a safe agent for skin lightening. Its use was banned in over-the-counter cosmetic skin-lightening products by the European Union in 2000. This is because it became apparent it was being used on much larger areas of skin and for longer periods than deemed safe. It should only be obtained by prescription, though alarmingly a quick search of the internet shows it can be bought online and I would strongly recommend against this risky practice as there is no certainty of product purity.

b) Natural active ingredients

Kojic acid: This is derived from a fungal species and has a long history in Asia as a skin-lightening agent. Concentrations of 1–4 per cent are needed for response and products should be used twice daily for two months. It is often used in combination with other agents such as arbutin, glycolic acid, liquorice extract and vitamin C. Products worth trying include Mario Badescu Whitening Mask and Sesderma Kojicol Plus Skin Lightener Gel.

Glabridin (liquorice extract): The main active ingredient in liquorice extract is 10–40 per cent glabridin. It is also often found in combination with other skin lightening agents such as arbutin, kojic acid, vitamin C and mulberry extract. There are various glabridin products on the market, including Ren Radiance Perfection Serum and Neostrata Enlighten Pigment Lightening Gel.

Arbutin: This is extracted from the bearberry plant and needs to be used in concentrations of at least 1 per cent in products for any lightening effects. Try iS Clinical White Lightening Complex, Eve Lom Brightening Cream and The Ordinary Alpha Arbutin 2% + HA.

Niacinamide: Niacinamide (vitamin B3) has a number of effects when used in creams and gels. It will regulate oil production and act as an anti-inflammatory agent, but also can be used for skin brightening. Personal favourites include The Ordinary Niacinamide 10% + Zinc 1% and Paula's Choice Resist 10% Niacinamide Booster.

Soy: Natural soybeans contain a protein that can interact with the melanin pathway and has been used in moisturizers to even skin tone. The active protein is degraded with pasteurization so the effect will only be found in fresh soy milk.

Vitamin C: Topical vitamin C interferes with pigment production, but not all forms of the vitamin (and there are many) are effective at the physiological level. If possible, opt for products that contain magnesium ascorbyl phosphate (MAP), ascorbyl-6-palmitate, disodium isostearyl 2-o-L-ascorbyl phosphate and ascorbic acid sulphate. Vitamin C is unstable and often combined with soy and liquorice for depigmenting effects. Concentrations of up to 20 per cent are ideal; any higher than this will cause significant irritation. Products to look out for include Obagi: Professional-C Serum, The Ordinary Magnesium Ascorbyl Phosphate 10% and Skinceuticals C E Ferulic.

Glycolic acid: This is derived from sugar cane and has important skin-lightening effects. It comes in varying strengths and there are multiple over-the-counter creams, cleansers and toners, usually containing 4–10 per cent glycolic acid; these include Pixi Glow Tonic Exfoliating Toner, Vichy Idealia Peeling, Jan Marini Bioglycolic Face Cleanser and Neostrata Foaming Glycolic Wash.

Glycolic acid can also be used as a medical-grade chemical peel, only available in clinic, in higher concentrations of 30–70 per cent. It should ideally be started at low concentrations and built up to avoid skin irritation, particularly in pigmented skin. Glycolic acid works well in combination with hydroquinone as the acid enhances hydroquinone penetration through the skin layers.

Azelaic acid: This has a number of uses and can treat rosacea and acne. In concentrations of 15–20 per cent twice daily for six months, it can also improve pigmentation. Azelaic acid is available on prescription, although there are weaker preparations available over the counter, such as The Ordinary Azelaic Acid Suspension 10% and Paula's Choice Clear Skin Clearing Treatment.

Retinoids: These have been shown to have some activity in reducing the pigmentation associated with melasma. Tretinoin is the most effective of these, and is often used in combination with hydroquinone, but is only available on prescription. There are weaker versions, such as retinol creams, available over the counter; try The Ordinary Retinol 1% and Medik8 Retinol 10TR Serum.

The suggested melasma treatments above are all options to trial at home; if, however, you have been using these for at least three months with no obvious improvement, it is a sign that medical intervention may be necessary. These are coming up next.

c) Clinical treatments

Chemical peels: Chemical peels are discussed in more detail in chapter 7, 'Anti-ageing Treatments'. They have a number of uses including skin resurfacing and treatment of pigmentation. For anyone of my generation, chemical peels will conjure up images of Samantha from *Sex and the City* and her raw, red face. In reality, chemical peels are a really good way of treating specific skin concerns and, in my experience, produce some very good results for pigmentation; they rarely disappoint me.

Chemical peels are a generic term for a large number of ingredients that can potentially be applied to the skin to cause exfoliation and skin shedding. Peels come in varying depths depending on the skin layer that needs targeting.

The process of having a peel usually takes about twenty minutes. The skin is first cleansed and then a chemical solution is applied to remove skin cells and stimulate growth of new, healthy skin. There may be a feeling of tightness or stinging when the peel is applied. It is left in contact with the affected area for minutes to hours depending on the agent. Typically, with most chemical peels for melasma, there can then be redness, peeling and shedding of skin for up to seven days until new skin comes through.

After a peel, it is really important to be careful with sun exposure and wear high factor SPF (minimum 30, ideally 50) for at least four weeks afterwards. The skin is new and more vulnerable to damage from UV than before the peel took place. There is a high risk of pigmentation returning quickly, possibly worse than pre-treatment if care is not taken.

Common agents used for peeling in melasma include salicylic acid, glycolic acid, trichloroacetic acid (10–30 per cent) and tretinoin. Some peeling agents contain a mixture of brightening agents and acids for best results.

There is a risk with chemical peels of either no response, potential worsening of pigmentation, infection and scarring. It goes without saying, then, that you should always seek the advice of a qualified dermatologist who is able to offer and perform a variety of peels (and have the skill to offer laser treatments if necessary).

Laser: Laser treatments in melasma remain a controversial topic, mainly as laser can produce unpredictable results and potentially cause worsening of pigmentation. For those that are interested, there are a number of different types of laser that have been used for melasma including the Q-switched (QS) Nd:YAG, dual yellow laser (again, don't be afraid of the technical-sounding names!), 755nm Alexandrite and 1550nm fractional laser. Laser energy often needs to be reduced to prevent inflammation in the epidermis that can trigger worsening of pigmentation. In addition to laser, some light devices such as intense pulse light (IPL) may also be used.

There remains a role for laser treatments, which can often be combined with peels and topical therapies for best results. Often, a course of treatment is required to fade stubborn melasma.

When choosing a practitioner, it is important to find someone that has knowledge about all potential treatment options and is able to use most, if not all, methods described. If you suffer from melasma and have ethnic skin, again, care needs to be taken to find someone that has experience in dealing with darker skin types.

Tranexamic acid: There is data which suggests that tranexamic acid, either injected into the skin or taken orally (250mg twice daily), may have a role to play in melasma treatment. This is not, as yet, considered a standard treatment, as taken orally the drug can slow the breakdown of blood clots; in some people this has the potential to lead to thromboses and other clotting complications.

Prevention

Sunscreen remains the cornerstone of prevention for melasma. There is plenty of scientific evidence showing that ultraviolet light from the sun (UVA and UVB rays) can drive this condition and make it worse. More recently, there is also data implicating visible light in the development of melasma and pigmentation in darker skin types.

The ideal sunscreen is therefore of high factor, SPF 50, with protection against UVA, UVB and high-energy visible light. Good options include Heliocare 360 gel. Alternatively, a mineral sunscreen containing zinc or titanium with an SPF 50 is suitable. This needs to be worn daily as part of regular skincare for melasma patients.

AGE SPOTS (FRECKLES, SOLAR LENTIGINES, 'LIVER SPOTS')

Brown spots and discolouration commonly develop in sun-exposed sites of fair-skinned people. They can, however, also occur in those who tan easily or have darker skin. Typically, they are found on the face, chest, forearms and the backs of the hands. They become more prominent as time passes and one gets older, and are the result of cumulative sun exposure over the years. Affected areas are not necessarily symmetrical and may be patchy or scattered. Sometimes there are other associated signs of sun damage, such as lines, wrinkles or 'crepey' (like crepe paper) skin. It is not usually considered a chronic condition and often responds well to treatment.

Treatment

Treatment strategies to make age spots fade are very similar to melasma treatments.

a) Creams and gels

Retinoid and hydroquinone creams and gels are commonly used to fade marks. This can take up to three months before any benefit is noticed. Prescription tretinoin is the gold standard and has a wealth of scientific support for its effectiveness. There are, nevertheless, useful over-the-counter products to try, which include The Ordinary Retinol 1% and Retriderm Max Vitamin A Ultra 1.0% Retinol Skin Serum.

b) Cryotherapy

Solitary or a few scattered age spots can be frozen away in a matter of seconds with a treatment of liquid nitrogen at a temperature of -196°C. It feels cold and sore and the affected areas have the potential to blister over the following few days, and may settle with an area of pale pigmentation compared to the surrounding skin. I should stress that this procedure should only be carried out by a qualified practitioner, such as a dermatologist or trained GP, but is perfectly safe and a very common treatment.

c) Chemical peels

The same peels discussed above for melasma can also be used to tackle age spots.

d) Light and laser

IPL is one of the most common treatments and consists of a gentle light beam. It is used for its ability to fade age spots over the face and chest. Often, a course of three to six sessions may be required depending on severity and response. Treatments are carried out at four to six weekly intervals and take about twenty to thirty minutes to treat the full face. The treatment is not painful but feels like intermittent hot elastic bands flicked against the skin. Care must be taken with sun protection following the treatment and for one month afterwards. Treated skin can be red for up to a day and there may be mild swelling for a few days.

Lasers can also be used to treat age spots. These include the QS Nd:YAG, QS-Ruby, 1550nm/1927nm (also known as Fraxel Dual) or ablative lasers such as an Erbium:YAG or carbon dioxide. Always enquire about the type of laser treatment your dermatologist is recommending for you, and why that specific choice has been made.

Prevention

Age spots develop mainly as a result of sun exposure, so it goes without saying that sun protection is key in prevention. If treatments are carried out, it is important to use high factor afterwards (SPF 30–50 is recommended) in the same way as one would for melasma treatments.

Many patients have annual maintenance treatments such as peels or IPL to keep any newly forming age spots at bay.

DARK EYE CIRCLES

Dark eye circles (periorbital hypermelanosis or periorbital hyperpigmentation) are another commonly encountered condition that presents to dermatologists. It affects both eyes and typically the lower eyelid skin. Those who have this condition often feel they look excessively tired, hungover or sad.

Causes

Dark eye circles can develop for a number of reasons. It tends to be more common in ethnic skin types, those with a genetic predisposition and increasing age. It can, however, be the result of other skin problems (e.g. allergy, eczema, melasma) or medical issues (e.g. thyroid disease, hay fever).

Prominent circles can be the result of excessive pigmentation in the skin, loss of fatty tissue in the eyelid or around the eye, puffy eyelids, thinning of the skin and prominent shadowing due to skin laxity. Whilst these factors are partly controlled by one's genetics, other factors such as ageing, smoking, fatigue, dehydration and even menstruation can also have a part to play.

Treatments

As there are a number of potential causes of dark eye circles, it is worthwhile to be assessed first by either your family doctor or dermatologist so that other medical causes can be ruled out.

There are a number of treatment options available to treat dark eye circles but the honest truth is that it can be challenging and often one treatment is not enough; a course can be required. In addition to this, different treatment types are usually needed in the same individual to produce significant results.

Lifestyle factors

Before jumping straight into medical treatments, there are a number of lifestyle factors that can be addressed which may help.

- Make sure you are getting enough sleep each night; for most people this should be about eight hours. Poor-quality sleep or lack of sleep can worsen eye circles.
- Your diet should be healthy, limiting alcohol and salty foods. These can cause dehydration and puffiness, making dark circles more prominent.
- Ultraviolet light (always to blame!) can make pre-existing dark circles worse, so high-factor SPF designed for the eye area (e.g. Skinceuticals Mineral Eye UV Defense SPF 30) is an absolute must on a daily basis.

- It is equally as important to invest in a good-quality pair of sunglasses that carry a CE mark (this means that they reach a certain EU standard of quality). A good retailer or your regular optician will be able to advise on this if there is any doubt on your purchase.

Camouflage

Not everyone may wish to proceed to medical treatments that can be invasive, and for some people simply covering up dark circles is enough. Products that are applied need to be waterproof, have holding power and provide high coverage. Colour correctors can be helpful before product application. Pink and peach tones will help neutralize darkness and visible veins in fair skin; orange and red tones can help darkness in deeper skin tones. For a natural result, these need to be blended. There are a large number of good under-eye concealers available on the market and choice mainly comes down to your own preference. Personal recommendations include MAC Studio Finish SPF 35 Concealer, NARS Creamy Concealer and Dermablend Smooth Liquid Camo Concealer.

Medical treatments

a) Creams and gels

For the majority of people, the most convenient way to treat dark eye circles is with the application of topical creams or agents. Many of these have limited scientific trials to back their use, but from personal experience I would say they are effective in reducing the amount of pigment or melanin in the skin, as well as improving the appearance of darkness, shadows or pigmentation. A number of agents can be used, often in combination.

When looking for over-the-counter brightening agents, products that contain the following ingredients can be helpful:

- vitamin C (magnesium ascorbyl phosphate, sodium ascorbate)
- arbutin
- kojic acid
- soy
- liquorice extract
- mulberry extract
- aloesin

- niacinamide
- azelaic acid
- retinol

Prescription products are likely to contain hydroquinone (2–4 per cent) and retinoids. These have the ability to produce irritation around the delicate eye area, and therefore use should be built up gradually under the guidance of a dermatologist.

b) Chemical peels

Chemical peels are often used to treat a variety of facial pigmentation problems including melasma and age spots as discussed previously. Deep peels should be avoided in the under-eye area due to the risk of scarring and worsening of pigmentation, but a course of light peels can help to some degree over time. Commonly used peels in this area include trichloroacetic acid (TCA) 3–6 per cent, lactic acid, mandelic acid and glycolic acid. They result in mild skin shedding over the course of a few days, but normal activities can be resumed quickly.

c) Microneedling

Microneedling is a minimally invasive skin procedure which uses a device with small needles to make
tiny punctures in the skin. It is not painful as it is
performed after the application of numbing cream.
This can often be combined with chemical peels, as
microneedling will increase the penetration and
therefore activity of the peel. There will be redness
and swelling after the procedure which can take
a few days to settle, as the skin around the eye area
is thin.

Combining microneedling with another procedure known as platelet-rich plasma (PRP) therapy
has also gained popularity for dark eye circles, but
the scientific evidence for this is limited. PRP hit
mainstream media after Kim Kardashian posted
photos of her 'vampire facial' for facial rejuvenation
on social media. A blood sample is taken and then
placed in a centrifuge. Plasma rich in platelets and
growth factors is extracted and then placed on to the
skin after microneedling. Often, more than one
treatment is required and results are variable.

d) Lasers

Lasers which target pigment, such as the QS-Ruby, QS-Alexandrite and 1064 Nd:YAG can be used as well as the 1550nm Fraxel. Laser treatments produce variable results, and often multiple courses are required. The eye is vulnerable to laser injury; treatments should only be carried out by an experienced practitioner. It is vitally important to have proper eye protection such as eye shields.

e) Dermal filler

If dark circles are due to the natural ageing process, which results in loss of fat underneath the eye, then small volumes of dermal filler – usually containing hyaluronic acid – can be injected or placed under the eye with a blunt device known as a cannula. Cannulas are gaining popularity for filler placement at this site as they are thought to be safer. Filler can smoothen out the skin and add volume, resulting in an improved appearance; this common filler treatment addresses 'tear troughs'.

There is a risk of swelling, bruising and bumps, and a theoretical risk of blindness. This latter complication is incredibly rare, however, and the procedure is very safe when done correctly by an experienced practitioner. The procedure is not permanent and depending on the product used the fillers are likely to last about twelve months.

Before you book to have this done, ensure you ask the person injecting you their training background and how many procedures they have carried out.

f) Fat transfer

If dark circles have developed due to significant loss of fat under the eyes, and there is marked hollowness as a consequence, then fat transfer can be an option (though it will not directly help the pigmentation). Fat can be taken from another body site and grafted or injected to the under-eye area. This should only be carried out by a plastic surgeon.

Treating dark eye circles is complex and requires patience. Multiple sessions and combinations are required, and often it is a case of trial and error to see what works best. The key is to see a knowledgeable cosmetic dermatologist with access to a range of treatments, who can assess the underlying cause of dark circles before initiating a treatment plan.

6

LIFESTYLE

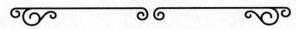

SLEEP

Having healthy skin goes hand-in-hand with having a healthy mind and body. Whilst we are unable to change our genetics or the hand we have been dealt in life, controlling environmental and lifestyle factors is firmly within our grasp. Life is about balance and self-care; we owe it to ourselves to look after what we have, for the relatively short duration of time that we are here.

When it comes to your skin, getting enough sleep is one of your basic beauty commandments. This has been echoed over the years by well-meaning older relatives, magazines and bloggers. And they are all absolutely correct. Sleep is a fundamental human requirement. During my twenties, there is no doubt I abused my sleep–wake cycles. Now, closer to forty, I give myself eight hours of sleep most nights of the week. I appreciate I am in a fortunate position to be able to do this; it would be much harder if I was still doing shift work, worked late into the evenings or had small children.

The concept of 'beauty sleep' is not a new one. Experimental studies have demonstrated that lack of sleep can make individuals look less healthy, less attractive and more tired. Studies aside, it's not rocket science to see that sleep deprivation can worsen under-eye circles and cause sallow, dull skin.

Skin is a dynamic organ, and provides an interface between the body and external environment. What our skin endures during the day is very different from what it faces at night. Think about it. We are at much higher risk of physical injury, exposure to ultraviolet radiation and microbes, as well as temperature extremes to name a few. So, naturally, it follows that the skin may work differently depending on the time of day.

We have long known that our body has a master biological clock found in the hypothalamus, a region of the brain. This clock establishes our circadian rhythm, the internal twenty-four-hour cycle coinciding with day and night. The circadian clock developed as life evolved on Earth; this was vital to protect us. Otherwise, we might be sleeping during the day and leaving ourselves vulnerable to attack. Our circadian clock dictates rhythmic changes in our physiology and behaviour. Many body processes have a circadian rhythm.

There is fascinating scientific work from the year 2000 onwards which demonstrates that skin cells have their own internal clock in addition to the brain's master clock. This includes many skin cell types; stem cells as well as cells that make collagen (fibroblasts) and pigment (melanocytes). These work together and in conjunction with the brain to produce rhythmic changes in the skin.

The skin's circadian rhythm affects nearly all of its functions. This includes skin hydration and water loss, oil or sebum production, blood flow, skin cell division and barrier function. These processes do not proceed at the same rate during the day and show peaks and troughs of activity. This is hugely important to understand for two main reasons. Firstly, it dictates when you should be using certain types of skincare treatment for best results. Secondly, chronic lack of sleep will disrupt your body's natural circadian rhythm, possibly through the generation of free radicals due to being metabolically active at unexpected times. This can lead to diminished barrier function of the skin and signs of accelerated skin ageing.

So what are some key changes in the skin during the day?

- Oil production peaks early afternoon and is lowest at night.

- Increased water loss through the upper skin layers (transepidermal water loss) at night.
- Skin barrier is more permeable at night.
- Many types of skin cells have a higher rate of division at night.

With this information in mind, you can now understand why my oily girl gang finds their make-up slips by the early afternoon. Even for normal skin types, many will start to get an oily T-zone after lunch. This is the time to be reaching for your blotting paper.

The skin loses more water content as we sleep compared to the day. This can be a problem for normal/dry skin types. After cleansing, it is worthwhile using a night cream if your skin is mature or dry. This is when your skin needs its extra moisture. For those with dry skin conditions such as eczema and psoriasis, it is even more important to ensure you moisturize before bed.

As the skin's barrier is more permeable at night and whilst we sleep, now is also the time to think about targeted treatments for your skin. This is the time to apply your treatment for stubborn spots, brightening agents for pigmentation and retinoids for anti-ageing. Conversely, individuals with sensitive skin types need to be cautious as products may penetrate more deeply.

Skin cells are busy dividing at night. Some studies show that cell proliferation is thirty times higher at night compared to midday. This process can be aided by adding alpha-hydroxy acids (e.g. glycolic acid, lactic acid) and retinoids into your skincare, which promote skin cell renewal and turnover. These are definitely worth considering if ageing or uneven skin tone is a concern.

There is no doubt that whilst we sleep the skin goes into a state of repair and regeneration. Other than optimizing your skincare routine to reflect this, getting enough sleep so that these processes can take place efficiently is vital. There is no fixed amount of sleep that an individual needs – it varies from person to person. Sleep requirements also change with age, with small children needing much more than adults. Experts agree that the average adult needs somewhere between seven and nine hours per night to rest the body and function effectively. This needs to be good-quality sleep without frequent interruption.

It is important to develop good sleep hygiene if you want to address the lifestyle factors that can impact your skin. Tips that can help develop a good sleep routine include:

Stress management: Feeling stressed or anxious is a common cause of sleep disruption. Whilst it is unrealistic to think we can get rid of all stress from modern-day life, coping mechanisms to deal with it are important. You need to find a method that works for you. Meditation, yoga and exercise may help.

Regular exercise: Regular physical exercise can improve sleep quality and duration. For some, but not all, high-intensity exercise in the evening one to three hours before bedtime can disrupt sleep, but this very much depends on the individual. If you find exercising at night keeps you awake, you are better off switching to early morning sessions instead. Low-impact exercise such as yoga and stretching before bed can still be helpful.

Stick to a sleep schedule: Try to go to sleep and wake up at the same time every day, including weekends and holidays. This helps set your body's internal clock and optimizes sleep quality.

Drink alcohol and caffeine in moderation: For those who are sensitive, caffeine can interfere with sleep for ten to twelve hours after its consumption. I had always suspected this was the case with me, but it was recently confirmed when I had some genetic testing carried out which showed that I was a slow caffeine metabolizer. With this in mind, I no longer drink coffee after midday. We all know that too much caffeine is a stimulant, so switch to your herbal teas instead. And for fellow green-tea lovers, remember this contains caffeine too!

Alcohol in excess can cause problems with sleep quality and quantity. Whilst it can initially help you fall asleep more quickly and deeply, it reduces rapid eye movement (REM) sleep. REM sleep is a vital part of the natural sleep cycle and its reduction can result in circadian rhythm disruption.

Avoid bright screens an hour before bed: Blue wavelengths of light emitted from bright screens like smart phones can cause all sorts of sleep disruption. And whilst a final check of your preferred social media before lights-out is tempting, it is far better for your health to avoid using them for at least an hour before bed. Blue light will increase alertness and it can take longer for you to fall asleep. This in turn will affect your natural circadian rhythm and REM sleep through a variety of mechanisms. Swap your phone for a good old-fashioned book to help you get to sleep.

Sleep remains a fundamental requirement for us to function. It is not a state of being where everything 'switches off' and shuts down. Rather, it is a highly active process with incredibly complex biological circuitry. Your skin relies on good-quality sleep to keep you looking rested and healthy, no matter what your age.

THE SKIN'S MICROBIOME

The human microbiome is a fascinating area generating much research and public interest. It was an area we knew relatively little about until fairly recent advances in next-generation sequencing technologies, which allow huge volumes of DNA in cells to be analysed rapidly. This has revolutionized our knowledge about the skin and its natural inhabitants.

The skin is a major interface between the body and its environment. In utero, or before birth, skin is sterile. After we are born, microbes rapidly start to colonize our skin; they form a complex ecosystem that lives alongside us. This includes bacteria, viruses and fungi. It is often said that in, and on, our bodies, microbial cells outnumber human cells by a factor of ten; we are more microbe than human! This set of microbes and their genetic material are our 'microbiome'.

The human microbiome is diverse and shows variability between individuals; the unique combination on my skin is different from yours. It can also be influenced by factors such as age, sex, lifestyle, body site, occupation and disease.

Maintaining our skin microbiome is beneficial for our health. These 'good' microbes can prevent our skin being taken over by pathogenic or 'bad' ones. They also have a role to play in optimizing the immune function of the skin and influencing metabolic processes. Unsurprisingly, research shows that it is the outer protective barrier, or stratum corneum, that has the largest number of bacteria compared to other skin layers.

There are a number of resident bacteria that live on the skin. Certain body sites favour growth of one particular type over another; for example, sebaceous or oily areas such as the face and back have a different microbiome make-up than moist areas such as the armpits, which are different again from dry areas.

Skin microbiome research has become of interest due to growing recognition of its role in health and disease. Disruption in the microbiome may have a role to play in skin conditions such as acne and eczema. Being able to manipulate the microbiome can potentially provide us with exciting new methods to treat skin problems.

Acne

Sebaceous areas such as the face contain high proportions of the bacteria *Propionibacterium*. In particular, *Propionibacterium acnes* (*P. acnes*) has been linked to the development of acne.

P. acnes is a bacterium that can be found on everyone's skin. However, in those who have acne, certain strains of *P. acnes* are more common than in those without. This emerging data provides the potential opportunity of supplementing 'good' bacteria on to the skin that is able to counteract the troublesome culprits that lead to spots. Targeted treatments are undoubtedly better than using traditional antibiotics, which simply kill all bacteria, both good and bad.

Eczema

Eczema is an extremely common condition and thought to affect nearly 20 per cent of children in the Western world. It has become more common over the decades, possibly related to an environmental component. The 'hygiene hypothesis' suggests this may be due to reduction in family size and increase in personal hygiene and cleanliness. We are not exposed to dirt and microbes in the same way as we were in the past, which in turn may have affected our skin's microbiome.

Many of those suffering from eczema have the bacterium *Staphylococcus aureus* on their skin. Studies have shown that during a flare-up of eczema, there is an increase in *Staphylococcus aureus* bacteria but, intriguingly, a concurrent reduction in the other types of bacteria on the skin, i.e. a reduction in bacterial diversity. This is of huge interest; it prompts the fascinating question of whether supplementing a 'normal' microbiome from a non-eczema sufferer can prevent flare-ups.

Skin microbiome research is still in its early days. We do not have robust information as yet to understand how the microbiome can be manipulated to prevent or treat skin problems. The beauty world, however, is always quick to spot potential and probiotic skincare is becoming more widely available.

Probiotic skincare

The World Health Organization defines probiotics as 'live microorganisms which, when administered in adequate amounts, confer a health benefit on the host'.

Oral probiotics for gut health have been around for quite some time and two of the best-known probiotic bacteria are *Lactobacillus* and *Bifidobacteria*. A question mark hangs over the benefit of oral probiotics in skincare. The resident gut microbiome is very different from the skin's natural fauna. What is right for the gut may not be right for the skin, even if we assume that the probiotic gets to the skin in high enough quantities following digestive processes.

Probiotic skincare, however, has gained much hype and interest. There are a number of beauty ranges that offer probiotic ingredients in their products and claim to provide a 'natural' or holistic approach, trying to correct the skin from within. They have become a bit of a buzzword in skincare but the real question is: do they work?

There are very few studies which show that certain probiotic agents when applied to the skin can help acne, redness and dry skin. These have been done on small numbers and the results are not always reproducible. However, that has not stopped the skincare market, and probiotic skincare is readily available should you choose to look for it, even from the large cosmetic houses.

Probiotic skincare relies on the theoretical premise that live bacterial cultures in their products can alter the skin's microbiome. Firstly, these cosmetic products, such as face creams, can create a protective barrier on the skin surface and prevent 'bad' bacteria from interacting with the skin. Secondly, some probiotics produce substances that can damage 'bad' bacteria, reducing inflammation.

These are the hypotheses anyway. Live bacterial cultures have a limited life span of a few days before they run out of a food source and die. Live cultures are therefore rarely used in cosmetic skincare. What *is* used more frequently is lysate; this is purified bacterial cellular material (e.g. bacterial cell walls, metabolites and dead bacteria). There is an assumption being made that lysate in skincare has the same biological effects as the live cultures.

Whilst the future for probiotics is bright in the health and beauty industry, one needs to be cautious in marketing a science that is still not fully understood. We still need more data on probiotic bacterial strains that may benefit the skin microbiome. To assume that products used for the gut will automatically help the skin in a cosmetic formulation is an error. I certainly remain sceptical, but open-minded. Having spoken to a number of cosmetic scientists and studied reviews of the data, I feel the evidence is lacking at present.

However, one day, hopefully in the not-too-distant future, microbiome research may allow us all to have a personalized approach to our skincare.

DIET

In the past decade, there has been a general drive to look after the skin in a more holistic manner. Focus has shifted to interest in prevention strategies. Reducing the likelihood of skin problems developing in the future has become just as important as their treatment.

There is no doubt that eating well and maintaining a good diet is essential for not only our general well-being, but skin health also. Glowing, lustrous, wrinkle-free skin is a common goal for many women and this is unlikely to be achieved by skincare alone. What you put inside your body needs the same care and thought as what you apply on the outside.

It has become fashionable in recent times for exclusion diets. So many patients I see are dairy-free, gluten-free or sugar-free for a variety of reasons. These can be related to gut health, skin, what their favourite celebrity or other social media influencer does, or simply the advice of a naturopathic doctor. Don't get me wrong, exclusion diets have a place; they are key, for example, for those that have genuine intolerances or allergies. But I think there are a large number of people that simply don't need to be cutting essential nutrients out of their diet. This is something that concerns me when I see patients who have been given poor advice and essentially been told to avoid eating nearly everything for the sake of their skin.

I firmly believe that balance is the key to a healthy diet. Personally, I am not in favour of cutting out food groups entirely and don't do diets of any description. The key is moderation and allowing occasional treats without beating yourself up about it. Too much of anything is a bad thing and the same logic applies to food.

So what should a healthy diet that has benefits for your skin look like? Well, the ideal diet aims to reduce inflammation and free radical damage in the skin. Antioxidants, minerals and other nutrients are needed to maintain skin integrity and act as co-factors to support biochemical processes in the body. Where possible, it is far better to get these from your diet in the form of whole foods than to take supplements.

Foods for healthy skin

a) Fatty fish

Salmon, mackerel and herring are rich sources of omega-3 fatty acids besides being naturally high in protein and zinc. Omega-3 fatty acids can be helpful in reducing inflammation in skin cells and may make your skin less sensitive to damage by UV radiation from the sun.

b) Fruit and vegetables

The antioxidants found in fruit and vegetables will neutralize damage by harmful free radicals in the skin. Vitamin C and E, beta-carotene, lycopene and lutein can offer some protection against damage generated by UV rays.

- Citrus fruits are a good source of vitamin C.
- Lycopene can be found in tomatoes.
- Sweet potato contains beta-carotene.
- Dark, leafy green and yellow vegetables contain lutein.
- Spinach and avocado contain vitamin E.

c) Nuts and seeds

Sunflower seeds are high in vitamin E and linoleic acid, a type of fat that can help skin hydration. Walnuts contain antioxidants such as vitamin E, essential fatty acids (which the body is unable to make) and minerals such as zinc and selenium. They should be consumed in moderation due to their high calorific content.

d) Green tea

Green tea contains compounds known as polyphenols which, when consumed regularly, can protect your skin from free radical damage from the sun. It may reduce the number of fine wrinkles and prominent blood vessels. It should not be consumed with milk.

e) Dark chocolate

Cocoa is high in antioxidants such as polyphenols and flavonoids. They can potentially improve blood flow to the skin and limit damage caused by the sun. Look for chocolate that is a minimum 70 per cent cocoa solids as anything with less is high in sugar. Again, moderating consumption is key.

So, a well-balanced diet is high in fish, olive oil, antioxidants, fresh fruit and vegetables, legumes, nuts and seeds. Conversely, there are a number of foods that should be limited in our diet. Sugar and refined carbohydrates, in particular, have been linked to acne and premature skin ageing. Acne and diet is discussed in chapter 5, 'Specific Skin Concerns'.

Sugar and skin ageing

There is a growing body of evidence which shows that sugar will contribute to premature skin ageing and inflammation by a process known as glycation. Sugar from dietary sources binds to proteins leading to the formation of harmful new molecules known as advanced glycation end products (AGEs). As these accumulate over time, they directly damage collagen and elastin, which give our skin its structural support. This process starts in one's mid-thirties and has a number of detrimental effects on the skin. It results in reduced skin elasticity, textural changes, wrinkles and skin sagging. The process by which AGEs form also results in free radical production, which can lead to further cell damage and inflammation.

Whilst there is much work to be done on the evolving science of nutrition and its effects on the skin, there are clearly basic principles that can be followed to maintain skin health. Many nutrients benefit the skin or prevent accelerated ageing through their antioxidant action or by serving as co-factors for key metabolic processes. It is important to develop and hone clean eating habits for overall improvement in general health and appearance.

EXERCISE

We all know that exercise is good for us. That regularly working out benefits our heart, lungs and mental health is hardly earth-shattering news. However, exercise and its effects on the skin – both good and bad – are often overlooked.

The biggest myth that reaches my ears (often after a hot yoga class) is how exercise and sweat are good for removing toxins from the body. Much to my concealed horror, this misconception is perpetuated time and time again. And often by medical professionals, who quite frankly should know better. There is no scientific evidence to suggest that exercise detoxifies the skin. Our amazing body is perfectly capable of getting rid of what we do not need. Our liver and, to a lesser degree, our kidneys are responsible for this task.

Nevertheless, exercise does have a number of positive effects on the skin. Regular exercise improves blood flow to skin cells. Blood will carry oxygen and vital nutrients where needed, whilst taking away waste products including free radicals that can damage the skin.

Exercise has also been demonstrated to reduce stress. Growing evidence shows that many inflammatory skin conditions (e.g. acne, eczema, psoriasis) can be aggravated by stress. Reducing stress levels with regular exercise may form part of a treatment or coping strategy in dealing with these conditions.

Exercise is also good for specific skin problems such as cellulite. Whilst cellulite is not life-threatening, it causes huge cosmetic concern for many women that I see. Maintaining a healthy body weight and increasing muscle mass can make the skin visibly more smooth and firm, reducing the appearance of cellulite. Incorporating a combination of high-intensity interval training and strength training will produce the best results.

Regular exercise can, however, also create problems with the skin and there are certain conditions that frequently require attention from a medical or cosmetic dermatologist.

Body acne

Body acne, often affecting the back, chest and sometimes the buttocks, is common in those who exercise frequently. Heat, sweat and occlusive clothing have the ability to block pores. Bacteria can then act on this to create spots.

A form of acne known as *acne mechanica* can also develop in those who do sport that requires wearing a helmet or backpack. Friction, occlusion, sweat and heat from raised body temperature combine to create spots.

The ideal solution to these problems is to shower immediately after exercise. Whilst it is tempting to sit around in gym wear, glugging down a juice, this is no good for your skin. The recent trend in 'athleisure' may also be contributing to the problem. If body acne persists, then switch to shower gels and body washes containing helpful ingredients such as salicylic acid, glycolic acid or tea tree oil; good ones include Murad Acne Body Wash, The Body Shop Tea Tree Skin Clearing Body Wash, Peter Thomas Roth Blemish Buffing Beads and Mario Badescu AHA Botanical Body Soap. Recurrent, ongoing, painful or deep spots or scarring should prompt medical attention as you may need stronger treatment.

If it is not possible to shower immediately, then get into the habit of keeping face wipes made for acne-prone skin (e.g. Garnier Pure Active 2-in-1 wipes) in your gym kit. After exercise, use these to wipe skin down until you are able to shower. It's not the ideal solution, but it is probably the next best thing.

Sun damage

Sunshine will put you at risk of developing a wide range of cosmetic and medical skin problems. These include premature ageing (sun spots, freckles, fine lines, wrinkles) and skin cancers such as melanoma. Whilst exercising and training outdoors has a number of health benefits, the biggest mistake I see is women failing to use sunscreen to protect their skin. The more vigilant will remember to apply SPF to their face, but neglect other parts of their exposed body. For example, many will train outdoors in shorts but fail to apply sunscreen to their legs. Considering that the commonest site for melanoma in women is the leg, it is definitely not a place to forget the SPF.

For those who are concerned about skin ageing, wearing regular SPF is equally as important. Ultraviolet light damages the skin leading to pigmentation, textural changes and wrinkles. If you are going to be outdoors then use a broad-spectrum sunscreen which offers UVA and UVB protection, and most people should aim for an SPF 30.

Infections

Communal showers, shared equipment and machines covered in sweat all work in perfect harmony to create an environment for your skin that predisposes it to picking up minor skin infections.

Viral warts and verrucae are caused by strains of the Human Papilloma Virus (HPV). These can be found on wet surfaces and easily penetrate the skin through small cuts or fissures. The same goes for fungal spores that are responsible for causing athlete's foot. Always wear flip-flops in communal showers and avoid going barefoot where possible to minimize the risk of infection.

Where possible, always wipe down gym equipment before use; do not assume this has been done already. Pay attention to small things. Do not expose any open cuts or wounds and wear a plaster to protect your skin if necessary. If, despite these measures, you pick up a gym infection, most of these can be sorted out by over-the-counter treatments. If problems persist, it is worthwhile seeing your GP or dermatologist for treatment.

Chafing

As you run, walk or jog, areas of friction, often where body folds meet and rub, can become inflamed or irritated. This is incredibly common, particularly if you carry a little bit of extra weight. In this situation, it is better to opt for appropriately fitted, low-friction fabrics. Using petroleum jelly or other lubricants on the areas prone to chafing can help. However, the truth is that it can still be hard to avoid.

Once chafing has developed, the skin needs to be looked after properly. After gentle cleaning, dry the area thoroughly and apply petroleum jelly. If the area is painful, red, swollen or scabby then seek medical advice as you may need an antibiotic ointment.

Now, don't let these common skin issues deter you from regular physical activity. Nearly every modality of exercise will boost circulation to the skin and reduce stress. Exercise should be incorporated as a lifestyle measure for healthy organ functioning, skin included.

POLLUTION

Air pollution in the UK is a huge problem. For many of us who live in towns and cities, pollution levels can cause a range of health issues. Whilst we have known about its effects on the heart and lungs for some time, it is now becoming apparent that our skin is also vulnerable to attack.

As skin is your outermost barrier, it is one of the first and largest targets for air pollution. So what exactly is air pollution? Air pollutants include the polycyclic aromatic hydrocarbons (PAH), volatile organic compounds (VOC), oxides, particulate matter, ozone and cigarette smoke. Prolonged and repetitive exposure to these agents can have negative effects on the skin.

Scientific studies in both animals and humans have shown that these components of air pollution can contribute to premature skin ageing (wrinkling, pigmentation spots) and worsening of inflammatory skin diseases such as eczema, psoriasis and acne. One major mechanism is via the generation of free radicals that can damage DNA in skin cells.

Short of leaving the city and moving to the countryside, what can you do to limit damage?

- Cleanse your skin every night to remove dirt and environmental toxins from the skin surface.
- Exfoliate once weekly (less if you have dry or sensitive skin) to give your skin a deeper clean. This will also improve the penetration of any products that are later applied to the skin.
- Use an antioxidant serum; antioxidants such as vitamin C and resveratrol have the ability to neutralize damage caused by free radicals generated by pollution.
- Use a regular sunscreen (minimum SPF 30). Don't forget that your skin also needs UV protection to help reduce the risk of skin cancers and signs of premature ageing.
- Moisturize daily, particularly if you have a tendency towards dry, inflammatory skin conditions (e.g. eczema and psoriasis). This will keep your skin hydrated, helping to maintain the integrity of the barrier function of your skin.

It has become fashionable over the last couple of years for creams to be marked as 'anti-pollution' as the air quality in our cities becomes ever worse. For many of us settled in city life, it is worth thinking about taking extra precautionary measures to protect against the noxious chemicals we are exposed to on a daily basis. We may not be able to control the environmental factors that lead to skin inflammation and ageing, but it is in our hands to try and limit their effects.

SMOKING

We are taught from a young age about the perils of smoking and its link with lung cancer. Cigarette smoking affects nearly every organ in the body, and your skin is not safe either. Smoking has been associated with premature skin ageing and wrinkles, poor or delayed wound healing and worsening of a number of skin diseases.

Premature skin ageing

The link between smoking and wrinkles has been known for many years. What's interesting is that women seem to be more susceptible to this than men. Smoking is associated with fine lines around the eyes ('crow's feet') and mouth ('smoker's lines'), which occur at an earlier age in smokers than in non-smokers.

Aside from early wrinkling, smoking causes a number of recognized facial changes. These include thinning of the skin, facial redness and prominence of the underlying bony contours of the face.

Whilst we don't fully understand how smoking exerts its negative effects on the skin, there are a number of proposed mechanisms. Smoking appears to activate enzymes which break down collagen and elastin fibres. It generates free radicals that can directly damage the DNA found in skin cells. Smoke also causes narrowing of blood vessels, thereby reducing blood flow to the skin; toxins can accumulate, resulting in subsequent changes to the supporting connective tissue.

Poor wound healing

There is a large number of scientific studies that demonstrate smoking will delay wound healing; this includes injury and wounds created by surgery. This is something to think about if you are considering a cosmetic procedure or having surgery for a medical reason.

Cigarette smoke exerts its action in a number of ways:

- Nicotine causes reduced blood flow soon after inhaling cigarette smoke. This results in reduced delivery of much-needed oxygen and other nutrients necessary for the skin to regenerate.

- Nicotine makes certain blood cells known as platelets more 'sticky'. Tiny clots can form, blocking small blood vessels, preventing oxygen reaching wound tissue. This lack of oxygen can also slow wound healing.
- Tobacco inhibits the activity of cells known as fibroblasts that are responsible for producing collagen. Collagen is needed for normal wound healing.

Smoking and skin disease

Smokers are at higher risk of developing a number of skin disorders. These include a type of skin cancer known as squamous cell carcinoma and other inflammatory conditions such as psoriasis, hidradentitis suppurativa and discoid lupus erythematosus.

The skin, like all other organs in the body, is susceptible to the damage caused by cigarette smoke. If you are a smoker, it may be time to consider kicking the habit and seek appropriate help if needed. Something to think about if you want to maintain your looks!

ALCOHOL

Now, I am definitely partial to a glass of white wine once or twice a week, but regular, heavy alcohol consumption can wreak havoc on your skin. Moderation, again, is the key.

Alcohol is a diuretic; as a consequence, it can dehydrate the skin. After a big night out, your skin will appear pale, sallow and less plump the following morning. Dehydration also prompts the body to cling to whatever water is present, often around the face, and can result in visible bloating.

Over time, redness and prominent facial blood vessels and visible broken capillaries appear. Many of those who suffer with skin conditions such as rosacea find that alcohol is one of their biggest triggers for redness and flushing or blushing.

Heavy drinking will deplete the body of vital nutrients and vitamins needed for healthy skin function. In particular, the body's stores of vitamins A, B, C and zinc are very vulnerable to this. Vitamins A and C are powerful antioxidants needed to neutralize free radical damage produced within the body and from external sources. Vitamin C is also needed for collagen production to provide the skin with support.

Sugary cocktails should be limited as sugar can drive a process known as glycation. Glycation results in sugar attaching to vital proteins like collagen in skin cells. This leads to the formation of harmful molecules, which can accumulate and contribute to premature skin ageing. For some, sugar can also drive acne so if you notice your skin is spotty after a heavy night, this could in part be the explanation.

The key to minimizing alcohol's effects on the skin is moderation and careful choice of drink selection. Colourless alcoholic drinks such as vodka, gin and silver tequila are probably better options than beer or cocktails laced with sugar. Remember to drink plenty of water during the course of the evening and before you go to bed, and rehydrate the following day. Eat lots of fresh fruit and vegetables to replace the nutrients you have lost. Resist the temptation to eat salty foods such as pizza and crisps that can contribute to water retention in the wrong body sites. Your skin will thank you for it in both the short and long term.

7

ANTI-AGEING TREATMENTS

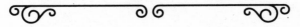

Standards of beauty, particularly for women, have always featured youth as a hallmark. As time passes, we all start to worry about the effects of the natural ageing process – the wrinkles, loose skin, sagging and uneven skin tone. Many of us embrace the changes that added years bring to our lives and seek no intervention, but I also see many patients in clinic who feel that the visible signs of ageing do not match how they feel on the inside. I think it is pretty safe to say that the anti-ageing market is booming and shows no signs of slowing down.

We women are leading very different lives from those of our mothers and grandmothers. We have successful careers, financial independence and often choose to have children at a later age than generations before. Life expectancy for the population is also increasing. The idea of 'middle age' has shifted and these factors may contribute to a discrepancy between internal and external self-perception. Mass media and advertising promote an idea of beauty and youth that is difficult, if not impossible, to attain without any extra help. Not everyone is genetically blessed.

And it is not just women in their forties and over that this affects. Of interest, there is data from recent years showing that women between the ages of twenty and thirty are increasingly opting for cosmetic interventions. From personal experience, the enquiries in my practice reflect this trend. We live in the age of the 'selfie', millennials engage in social media from an early age and information is more accessible than it has ever been. It is easy to follow celebrities on Instagram and see what procedures they are having done to maintain their looks.

Many may choose to 'age gracefully' and have no interventions. For most people, there is curiosity about what could be done coupled with fear of unnatural-looking results (the media has an unhealthy obsession with 'botched' procedures) and being judged by others as vain. The truth is simply that most of us lie on a spectrum of what we feel comfortable doing to our face and body. For some, having Botox and dermal fillers is part of the same maintenance and upkeep as threading their eyebrows or colouring their hair. For others, their comfort zone lies with having non-invasive treatments such as laser, but they would not dream of having injections. Neither is wrong or should be judged; only you can decide where on this spectrum you lie and what is right for you.

One thing I will add is that cosmetic interventions done well should not be obvious and should simply exist to enhance what is already there. Treatments should not try to make a fifty-five-year-old look twenty-five; they are there to make a fifty-five-year-old look good for her age, but not necessarily younger. On a personal note, I am not a fan of the overdone, unnatural look I often come across in the media – the over-inflated cheeks, over-filled lips and frozen foreheads.

CREAMS AND GELS

The elixir of youth has yet to be bottled and sold. Despite impressive marketing and celebrity endorsements, very few creams, gels and serums have robust data behind them for anti-ageing. I hate to be the bearer of bad news but creams will not help skin sagging or laxity. These changes occur due to loss of volume of fat and bone under the skin, which happens to all of us as time passes. No topically applied cream can replace that.

That said, there is science to show that some aspects associated with ageing can be helped by creams. Certain agents can be used to reduce pigmentation, fine lines and wrinkles, and slow down the signs associated with skin ageing. These include retinoids, antioxidants, botanicals and sunscreen. Anti-ageing strategies are very much focused on limiting long-term damage from sunlight, which is the most significant factor in skin ageing.

Retinoids

The retinoid family consists of a group of compounds that are derived from vitamin A. These have been available in skincare since the 1970s and are the only topical agents that repeatedly demonstrate anti-ageing effects in scientific studies. Retinoids are able to minimize the appearance of wrinkles, slow the breakdown of collagen and fade pigmentation or age spots. They work by improving skin cell renewal and stimulating collagen production.

Retinoids are a firm favourite of both dermatologists and beauty editors alike. There are a large number available, all marketed for their anti-ageing properties, but the truth is that they are not all the same in their effects. Getting the right retinoid for your skin is a minefield, given the sheer number of options available on the market. So how do you know which one to buy? Are the prescription-strength ones better than the ones you can buy over the counter?

Let's start with looking at individual ingredients. Retinyl esters, retinol, retinaldehyde, adapalene, tretinoin, isotretinoin and tazarotene are all different types of retinoid. Lots of names, but all are slightly different compounds. The key, however, is that your skin is only able to use a retinoid in the form of retinoic acid to get clinical benefit. While prescription tretinoin and isotretinoin are already retinoic acids, the conversion process of the other noted ingredients takes place in the skin. Retinyl esters are converted to retinol, then retinaldehyde, then retinoic acid. So a retinol-containing product is firstly converted into retinaldehyde and then retinoic acid, i.e. a two-step process. Products that require the fewest conversion steps tend to be more effective for anti-ageing purposes.

a) Over-the-counter retinoids

- Retinyl esters
- Retinol
- Retinaldehyde
- Adapalene (previously a prescription-only agent but has become available over the counter for the treatment of acne)

b) Prescription-only retinoids

- Tretinoin (retinoic acid)
- Isotretinoin (synthetic retinoic acid)
- Tazarotene

Most of the initial scientific studies looking at skin ageing and retinoids were carried out with tretinoin (retinoic acid). Tretinoin was found to be twenty times more potent than retinol. However, even 1 per cent retinol has been shown to be effective at twelve weeks in improving fine lines and wrinkles.

If prescription-strength tretinoin is more effective, then why do we bother with the other agents? Well, this largely comes down to tolerability. The more potent the retinoid, the higher the likelihood it will cause problems with skin irritation, such as burning, stinging, redness and scaling. There is a trade-off between clinical benefit and potential side effects.

So if you are looking for a suitable over-the-counter retinoid product, choose one that contains either retinol or retinaldehyde. These are likely to be more effective than the retinol derivatives such as retinyl acetate, retinyl propionate and retinyl palmitate. There are many good non-prescription-strength products available but it is important to do some detective work and check the active ingredients; simply being advised it is a retinoid and therefore anti-ageing is not enough if you want results. Wasting hard-earned time and money is avoidable if you do your homework but once you have found the correct product, it is worth making a retinoid part of your anti-ageing armoury.

Here are some pointers for the next time you're at your favourite skincare counter.

What should I buy? Over-the-counter products containing retinol or retinaldehyde. If buying a retinol product, check that it contains a minimum concentration of 0.1 per cent.

When should I start using these? From your late twenties onwards.

What's the best way to use them? Retinoids are best used at night after cleansing the skin; a small pea-sized amount should be adequate. It can take three to six months of regular use before any improvement in the skin will be seen. If the skin feels dry or tight, moisturizer can be applied twenty to thirty minutes later.

Are there any side effects? Retinoids can initially cause redness and irritation, so it may be wise to gradually build up use, from two to three times a week to every night if your skin will tolerate it. Skin treated with retinoid is sensitive to ultraviolet radiation and at risk of burning; sunlight also makes the product less effective. Night-time retinoid use should be combined with daily regular broad-spectrum sunscreen of at least SPF 30 during the day to mitigate these effects.

Antioxidants

Antioxidants have been the new big thing for a few years now. It is hard to avoid coming across the word all the time in food and skincare.

So what are antioxidants? An antioxidant is simply a molecule that prevents the oxidation of other molecules. Their benefit is that they block the damage caused by free radicals and reactive oxygen species.

Free radicals are molecules or atoms with an unpaired electron. Having an unpaired electron makes the atom or molecule more chemically reactive. In addition to free radicals there are other oxygen species (e.g. hydrogen peroxide, hypochlorite ion) that are also highly reactive. Free radicals and reactive oxygen species are able to cause irreversible and destructive changes to proteins, DNA and lipids (fats) found in cells and tissues. They are generated by exposure to UV radiation from the sun (the leading cause of external skin ageing) and by certain biological processes in the body that generate energy.

There are a number of antioxidants available in skincare products whose role is largely to prevent oxidative damage to the skin rather than treat the signs of ageing once they have developed. Antioxidants are highly unstable molecules which break down quickly, rendering them inactive. As such, antioxidant products need to be formulated very carefully to ensure that they remain effective.

Antioxidants to look out for in skincare products:

- Vitamin C
- Vitamin E
- Resveratrol
- Grape seed
- Green tea
- Silymarin from milk thistle
- Coffeeberry

a) Vitamin C

Vitamin C has a number of roles in skincare. It is an antioxidant, skin-brightening agent and anti-inflammatory, and is also required for the synthesis of collagen, which gives our skin its support structure. It should be used for skincare in concentrations of up to 20 per cent. Higher percentages can potentially cause irritation.

There are a number of vitamin C derivatives available on the market and not all are equally effective. Look out for these more stable chemical forms of vitamin C:

- Magnesium ascorbyl phosphate
- Ascorbyl-6-palmitate
- Disodium isostearyl 2-o-L-ascorbyl phosphate
- Ascorbic acid sulphate
- Tetraisopalmitoyl ascorbic acid

Vitamin C has an excellent safety profile and can be used in conjunction with other anti-ageing treatments such as retinoids, sunscreen and other antioxidants. It has been shown to protect the skin from sunlight by reducing free radical damage by

UV radiation and should be used in the morning before sunscreen application.

A common misconception about vitamin C is that oral supplementation will help the skin. The truth is that when vitamin C is taken orally, it has relatively little bioavailability in the skin (meaning that only a small proportion of it actually gets to the skin after it is metabolized in the gut). Applying it straight to your skin is therefore much more effective.

b) Vitamin E

Vitamin E is commonly known as tocopherol and the most widely used form is alpha-tocopherol acetate. Tocopherol and its commonly used forms are oils so high doses can often be greasy or sticky on the skin. Vitamin E has been shown in studies to reduce the number of sunburn cells and limit the potential damage associated with UVB radiation from sunlight. Cream containing 5–8 per cent vitamin E can also help with signs of ageing due to the sun, such as reducing fine lines. Using vitamin E and C together in skincare can increase their effects when compared to using them alone.

c) Resveratrol

Grapes, seeds, nuts and red wine are all sources of resveratrol (look for this in a product's ingredients list). When applied directly to the skin surface, it can limit damage caused by UVB radiation, according to some small studies. It has also been shown to improve skin firmness and elasticity at a concentration of 1 per cent. Due to resveratrol not being particularly water soluble, creating creams that hold it is difficult, and they can therefore be quite expensive. Unfortunately, you will not get the same benefits of resveratrol by increasing your red wine consumption!

Botanicals

There has been increasing interest in herbal-based products in the skincare, wellness and cosmetic arena. You will have seen more and more products being labelled as 'natural', containing 'natural oils' or coming from 'natural plant-based sources'. This is what we mean by 'botanicals'. Whilst some of these seem promising for skin ageing, the difficulty lies in the lack of scientific clinical trials to determine their true effectiveness.

There is no consistent definition of 'natural' in skincare products. This may come as a surprise but there is also no industry standard. There is little regulation or legislation covering the word's meaning and, sadly, it is essentially an often-abused marketing term making us believe we are not putting 'nasty chemicals' on our skin. The best bet is to start looking at the ingredients themselves rather than wholly relying on a product labelling itself as natural. Ingredients are listed in descending order of proportion of content, so if you are looking for natural skincare, ensure that the synthetic agents appear lower down the list.

Organic skincare is another interesting area. Product claims are not specifically regulated under current European Union law. There are varying standards of definition between organizations leading to much confusion and lack of consistency. Organic products should be those that are made of ingredients found in nature. They should be free of synthetic chemical use in both the field and production process. In the US, products can claim to be organic if 95 per cent of their components are organic and can be labelled as organic-derived if 70 per cent of their ingredients are organic.

Simply because a product is labelled as natural or organic does not mean it is necessarily safe. Skin reactions and sensitivity are still possible with these ingredients. For example, studies have shown that Chinese herbal preparations applied to the skin can cause skin reactions such as dermatitis, liver problems and birth defects if used during pregnancy in up to 30 per cent of people.

One of the difficulties in trying to study botanical or herbal treatments is that they are more susceptible to quality variation than their synthetic counterparts. Numerous factors such as health of the plant, harvest time, transport, processing and extraction methods need to be taken into account. Whilst there is no doubt credible research is required, however, there is growing data around certain botanicals. But it is important not to fall into the trap of buying 'snake-oil' products with results based on pseudoscience.

Common botanicals used in anti-ageing products in their topical form include coffeeberry, date palm kernel, oat, soy milk and total soy, glabridin, green tea, lavender, blackberry, goji, flax and mangosteen. These particular agents have been used in human clinical trials, albeit with small numbers of participants. There are many more used either in isolation or in combination with others. The bottom line is that robust data is needed and care needs to be taken to see through clever PR, branding and marketing. If you have a personal preference for botanical products, then

I'd steer you towards the ingredients I recommend above; however, if you want skincare supported by evidence-based science, a retinoid wins hands-down every time.

Peptides

Many of the face creams filling make-up aisles have contained peptides for many years now. They were one of the early ingredients in mass-market anti-ageing skincare and show no signs of going anywhere anytime soon. But what are they? And do they work?

So here is the chemistry part. Amino acids are the building blocks of peptides and proteins. Two or more amino acids linked in a chain form a peptide. A peptide chain of more than about a hundred amino acids forms a protein. Peptides are hugely important in the human body and often act as 'messengers', conveying information between cells and tissues.

Peptides are popularly claimed to repair the skin's extracellular matrix or scaffolding, thereby restoring its support structure and improving visible wrinkles. The most widely studied peptide in skincare is a pentapeptide (i.e. it has five amino acids), known as Pal-KTTKS. Let's take a look at this more closely.

Pal-KTTKS is a tissue-repair peptide known as a matrikine. It is essentially a small fragment of procollagen 1; this is a precursor in collagen synthesis in the skin. In lab studies, it has been shown to increase collagen synthesis in skin cells. In some small human trials, it was proven to thicken the skin and reduce fine lines and wrinkles, increasing levels of both collagen and elastin.

Does this mean we should be rushing out to buy products containing peptides? Well, not exactly. Yes, there is some supportive data, particularly of Pal-KTTKS. However, studies remain limited and small.

There are a huge number of peptides available in cosmetics and as our understanding of molecular cell biology increases, I have no doubt we will see more. They may well be an important method of improving skin appearance, but we need unbiased scientific data (ideally the data shouldn't come from the company that makes the product!) and more human studies. Much of our initial understanding came from trials in wound healing and investigations carried out in cell cultures – this does not always translate into a visible, positive benefit when tried out on the skin as a whole for anti-ageing purposes.

Pal-KTTKS often goes by the name 'matrixyl' on a product's ingredients list. Products on the market containing this include Olay Regenerist 3 Point Treatment Cream, Sarah Chapman Eye Recovery and No7 Protect and Perfect Intense Advanced Serum.

In conclusion, there is some supportive data for the use of peptides in anti-ageing skincare, but I would recommend caution in selecting the peptide you choose; at present, the best data is for matrixyl.

Growth factors

Skincare products containing growth factors remain controversial. In the human body, growth factors are proteins that regulate cell growth and division. Most of our knowledge about growth factors comes from their role in wound healing, but over recent years, skin creams containing growth factors are increasingly becoming commercially available.

Common growth factors used in skincare include:

- Epidermal growth factor (EGF)
- Vascular endothelial growth factor (VEGF)
- Transforming growth factor beta (TGF-b)

- Platelet-derived growth factor (PDGF)
- Keratinocyte growth factor
- Interleukins 6 and 8

Data from small studies suggests that growth factors used in combination may improve collagen production and improve the visible signs of ageing.

It all sounds good, but there are potential problems. Firstly, much of our knowledge on growth factors comes from wound-healing studies; wrinkles are clearly not the same as wounds. Secondly, growth factors do what they say – they encourage cell growth – and the question is, could this have an implication for formation of skin cancers or scar formation with prolonged use? Thirdly, growth factors are likely to work together in the body, not in isolation, which is often the way they are used in skincare. We simply do not have long-term safety data or robust clinical trials to definitely assess how useful they are in reality.

Sunscreen

This will always be the cornerstone of anti-ageing prevention. The sun remains the biggest cause of premature and accelerated skin ageing. Fine lines, wrinkling, uneven skin tone, pigmentation and textural changes occur because of damage from sunlight.

Sunlight contains a mixture of several different wavelengths of light. The main components are visible light, ultraviolet light and infrared radiation. Ultraviolet light, mainly UVA and UVB, is responsible for the majority of skin ageing. More recently, data is revealing that visible light and infrared radiation may also have more of a part to play in ageing than first realized due to the generation of free radicals in skin cells.

There are two main types of sunscreen: chemical and physical (mineral). Chemical sunscreens contain ingredients that behave as filters and reduce the level of UV penetrating the skin. They take approximately twenty minutes after application to become effective and should therefore be applied before going outdoors. Physical or mineral sunscreens are products that typically contain titanium dioxide and/or zinc oxide which physically block ultraviolet radiation, and work as soon as they are applied. Previously, formulations were chalky and thick but newer products rub into the skin much more easily. Mineral sunscreens are better for those with extreme sensitivity to UV radiation and sensitive skin.

From an anti-ageing point of view, sunscreen should therefore be worn on a daily basis. In the winter months, particularly in the northern hemisphere, using a moisturizer or make-up with SPF is satisfactory if you are going to be indoors during the day (although a separate sunscreen will still be better). In the spring and summer months, however, aim for a broad-spectrum sunscreen (i.e. one that offers protection against UVA and UVB) with an SPF 15–30 as a minimum. You do not necessarily need to get a separate sunscreen specifically for your face, but many body sunscreens are quite heavy and may not be suitable for blemish-prone facial skin. Facial sunscreens may also contain additional beneficial ingredients that body sunscreens lack.

Sunscreen that provides protection against visible light and infrared-A radiation is a bonus. Visible light and infrared generate free radicals, which can contribute to ageing. One of the current difficulties is that there is no universal labelling system for either of these. Using an antioxidant serum in conjunction with a standard sunscreen is therefore of value as it can neutralize the free radicals that the sun's rays generate. There are some products on the market that may provide full protection, often by incorporating antioxidants into their sunscreen formulations; these include:

- Heliocare 360 Oil-Free
- EltaMD Broad-Spectrum SPF 30
- Solero Facial Anti-Ageing Suncream SPF 30

In terms of product quantity, using approximately half a teaspoon of sunscreen for the face and neck is about right. The majority of us do not use enough sunscreen to get the factor on the bottle. It is important to ensure adequate application for the sunscreen to do its job for you.

Sunscreen is generally designed to last three years. However, if it has been exposed to extremely high temperatures, looks like it has changed in its colour or consistency or is past its expiry date then it should be discarded.

Common Sunscreen Myths

Does using an SPF of 30 provide double the protection of SPF 15?

Absolutely not. Firstly, **SPF** is only a measure of the **UVB** protection that a sunscreen provides. SPF 15 filters out about 93 per cent of UVB rays; SPF 30 will filter out 97 per cent. Of more interest, an SPF 50 filters 98 per cent of UVB. So as you can see, there is very little difference between using an SPF 30 and 50. Unless there is a history of skin cancer or light sensitivity, an SPF 15–30 is adequate for most of us. In the UK and Europe, UVA protection is normally designated by the letters UVA in a circle on the product label.

Is there any added protection if I use multiple products containing SPF?

Unfortunately not. If you use a moisturizer with SPF followed by sunscreen and then foundation with SPF it will not result in a greater effect. You will only have the protection of the highest SPF product that is being applied to the skin.

Do sunscreens cause cancer?

Current dermatological advice is that sunscreens are safe to use and do not increase the risk of cancer. The safety of sunscreens is nevertheless a topic frequently raised by my

238

patients during consultations. I have also certainly seen much online discussion on this subject centring on some of the ingredients in sunscreens such as retinyl palmitate, oxybenzone and nanoparticles.

Retinyl palmitate is a vitamin-A derivative found naturally in skin. Some studies have suggested that retinyl palmitate generates free radicals when exposed to ultraviolet (UV) radiation and that these can promote inflammation and cancer development in the body. However, the study often quoted to support this was carried out on hairless mice (which already have a higher risk of skin cancer) and retinyl palmitate was only studied in isolation. In real-life terms, when sunscreen containing retinyl palmitate is applied, antioxidants present in the body (e.g. vitamin C) will neutralize any free radicals that are generated. The current view from dermatologists is that there is no evidence that retinyl palmitate will cause skin cancer in humans.

Oxybenzone is a chemical filter found in sunscreens that is similar to oestrogen. There has been concern that it may interfere with hormone levels in humans. This has mainly come from a study in rats, carried out nearly fifteen years ago, where they were fed high levels of oxybenzone. There is a large difference between application of oxybenzone to human skin and oral consumption of oxybenzone in rats. Although oxybenzone can be absorbed by humans, it does not accumulate and is excreted. There is also no evidence to suggest that oxybenzone in sunscreens is dangerous to humans in the concentrations it is used.

Nanoparticles are very tiny particles (at the scale of a nanometre – one billionth of a metre). Physical sunscreens such as titanium dioxide and zinc oxide can be turned into nanoparticles; these make the resulting product smoother than the thick, white paste that results from using more granular minerals. Some fear that nanoparticles can be absorbed into the skin, causing damage. In actual fact, studies show that nanoparticles are only absorbed by the top layer of dead skin cells and not by living tissue. Additionally, the particles themselves have a tendency to clump together, so absorption rates are lower than expected. Evidence therefore suggests that nanoparticles are safe to use.

Are sunscreens waterproof?
Sunscreens cannot claim to be 'waterproof' but they can claim to be 'water resistant'. In actual fact, a sunscreen labelled 'water resistant' needs only to remain effective after forty to eighty minutes' exposure to wet conditions. What this means is that it is very important to reapply sunscreen after swimming or excessive sweating.

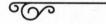

THE LAZY GIRL GUIDE TO ANTI-AGEING SKINCARE

Not everyone has the inclination or money to spend a great deal of time on their anti-ageing routine. The good news is that science really backs a small number of evidence-based products despite the plethora of options out there. Sunscreens and retinoids remain the backbone of any good anti-ageing regimen.

AM routine

- Cleanse
- Apply antioxidant serum
- Moisturize
- Apply sunscreen

PM routine

- Cleanse
- Apply retinoid

INJECTABLE TREATMENTS

Some people, despite getting their skincare just right, still feel the signs of ageing are catching up. Others, despite never having been meticulous about their skincare, are nevertheless also intrigued to know what else is on offer beyond simply using creams, lotions and potions (which are often heavily oversold and promise results that are simply not possible).

Visible signs of ageing can be improved with injectable treatments, most commonly Botulinum toxin injections (commonly known as Botox) and dermal fillers.

Botulinum toxin (AKA Botox)

Botulinum toxin is popularly known as Botox. In fact, Botox is a trade name for the active drug made by the company Allergan. There are other forms of Botulinum toxin including Azzalure and Bocouture available in the UK. Botox is the most popular and widely used and I shall refer to this, moving forwards, simply for convenience.

Botox has gained much popularity over the years and injectable treatments for this continue to rise year on year. I'm definitely seeing more people coming to me for Botox now compared to a few years ago. Its history is interesting and its use for cosmetic purposes was discovered entirely by accident. Botox was in use by eye doctors from the early 1980s to treat muscular disorders of the eye. It was noted incidentally that wrinkles around the eye were also disappearing following treatment and, by the end of the decade, Botox for cosmetic use had been born.

Botox is a synthetically made protein that is injected most commonly into the forehead, frown and eye area to treat wrinkles and lines at these sites. Its most basic action is to block nerve transmission to muscles causing temporary weakness. Wrinkles and lines become smoother or disappear altogether as a consequence.

Botox treatment can be used to treat wrinkles or lines in a variety of areas on the face. It will produce results that are simply not possible with creams. I've had it done a few times myself to treat very early frown lines (for which it's super-effective), and from a patient perspective found it quick and painless.

Common areas and lines that can be treated include:

Forehead lines: These lines develop over time, often due to repeated eyebrow raising. The affected muscle, frontalis, becomes overused and horizontal forehead lines develop. They can be visible from your twenties onwards. Botox injected into key sites in the forehead will soften these.

Frown lines: Frown lines, otherwise known as glabellar, or 'number 11', lines, are vertical creases that develop between the eyebrows. They occur due to repeated contraction of muscles known as the procerus and corrugator supercilii. Often, Botox injected into three to five sites in the frown area will treat these lines.

Crow's feet: Crow's feet occur due to the cumulative effects of smiling over the years; this is due to repeated contraction of the orbicularis oculi muscle, which encircles the eye. These become more prominent in your late twenties to early thirties and can also be effectively treated with Botox.

Botox also has a number of other aesthetic uses and can help with 'smoker's lines' around the mouth, jaw slimming and facial contouring, teeth grinding (bruxism) and treatment of excessive sweating (hyperhidrosis).

Botox injections do not work immediately and initial effects can be noted from between forty-eight to seventy-two hours later. Maximal effects are reached at about ten days and effects last on average three to four months. The treatments need to be repeated at regular intervals to maintain their effect. There is also an argument for using Botox in a preventative way. If injections are started before lines are present at rest, many people get out of the habit of frowning and permanent fixed lines may take longer to develop. This really needs to be assessed on a case-by-case basis, as caution is advisable before injecting those of a relatively young age.

There are potential side effects with Botox and it is important to go to an experienced practitioner who is able to show you other before-and-after photographs. In the UK, it is worth checking out the British Cosmetic Dermatology Group for practitioners (www.bcdg.info/practitioners) or finding a consultant plastic surgeon. In the US, make sure you choose a dermatologist or plastic surgeon that is board-certified; other parts of the world have similar accreditations.

The common side effects with Botox include bruising and swelling and a feeling of heaviness, but on rare occasions problems with a droopy eyebrow can occur with forehead injections. These are not permanent side effects and will wear off over time.

In truth, Botox is actually a straightforward and very safe procedure in the right hands. Many people come to me worried they will look overdone and frozen, or concerned their partner will notice if they have treatment. It is important to find a healthcare practitioner you trust and have a rapport with so you can explain exactly what you want of them. Choose a reputable clinic with good reviews and avoid places offering cut-price deals. Personally, I think it is all about subtle results, and all my patients have the option to come back and see me two weeks after their injections to make any small adjustments. In my experience, it is far easier to add more in two weeks; you can't take it out once it's in!

The injections themselves are done with fine needles and are not usually painful. They can cause some minor discomfort at worst, but nearly everyone tolerates Botox well without any problems. It is, however, still a medical procedure and a proper consultation should take place first including a thorough medical history.

Dermal fillers

As we age, collagen and elastin in the skin break down. At the same time, fat compartments lose volume and become thinner, particularly in the upper half of the face. The facial skeleton changes due to bone loss at strategic sites such as the mid-face and orbital bone around the eye. These factors combined together result in skin sagging, prominent skin creases such as nose-to-mouth lines (nasolabial fold) and jowl formation. This volume loss cannot be addressed by Botox and requires dermal fillers to fill or plump out the areas that have effectively become deflated. It is bad practice to treat individual areas in isolation (e.g. just the jowls); it is important to maintain balance and harmony in the whole face and so a complete facial aesthetic assessment should be carried out prior to any treatment.

There are many different types of dermal filler on the market including products that contain hyaluronic acid (e.g. Juvederm, Restylane), calcium hydroxylapatite (Radiesse), polycaprolactone (Ellansé) and poly-L-lactic acid (Sculptra). The vast majority of fillers now used are the hyaluronic acid varieties. These have increased in popularity over the years because they are non-permanent but long-lasting, cause few allergies and can be reversible and dissolved if necessary.

Before filler is injected, a medical consultation is necessary. Full facial assessment is vital to determine which areas require filling or volumizing. A thorough medical history and details of any medications or supplements should be taken first. Numbing cream can be applied for twenty to thirty minutes before injecting or ice can be used for numbing directly before the injections are placed. Results usually last for six to eighteen months depending on the product used.

Side effects include swelling, bleeding and bruising. Aspirin, ibuprofen and supplements such as vitamin E, fish oils, gingko biloba and ginseng should be discontinued as they can promote bleeding. Other potential problems include lumps, inflammation, filler migration to another site and infection. Certain areas are considered 'high-risk' sites such as the forehead, under-eye area and nose. There have been rare reported cases of blindness, so it is absolutely vital that the person you choose to inject you has been trained to the highest level in facial anatomy. Whilst the risks sound scary, in competent hands the procedure is safe.

Fillers have an excellent role in treating facial sagging, lines and even chin augmentation. I've had small volumes of strategically placed fillers to treat nose-to-mouth lines (nasolabial folds) which had become more noticeable around the age of thirty-five; the lower half of my face had started to look slightly heavy and even a bit saggy. I was pleased with the results of the filler. Whilst it may not be for everybody, I have no doubt I'll have more in the future.

The main problem with fillers is that their use is unregulated in the UK and consequently many in the industry feel they are a disaster waiting to happen. Unlike Botox, dermal fillers do not require a prescription, which means that anyone can theoretically buy and inject filler. This is hugely frightening when one knows the potential for things to go wrong. This puts the UK aesthetics industry in an interesting place. With its poor degree of regulation and little accountability for errors, it is all the more vital for the consumer to pick an experienced practitioner, in whose hands it is safe.

One thing that never ceases to amaze me is the number of aesthetic practitioners who themselves look rather odd as a result of their own overuse of injectable treatments – think big lips and 'chipmunk cheeks'. My personal feeling on this is that somewhere along the line, these individuals have lost their 'aesthetic eye' – that is, they are no longer able to perceive what is normal for a person's face. The purpose of these treatments should be to create natural results, not artificially enhanced or exaggerated features. I suspect that in many cases, this type of face is all such practitioners see on a daily basis, be it in their colleagues or their patients. This in turn may be driven by the pressures to appear 'young' that are prevalent in the industry but also sadly still intrinsic in our society, where it's fuelled by the unrealistic and unnatural body images all over social media.

You need to be confident that you are being given the best advice on any injectable treatments available, and sometimes the right answer is that it's not the right treatment for you. Practitioners should be sensitive to this, and give you an honest facial assessment. They should not automatically carry out a treatment just because they can.

I certainly have no qualms about saying no if I feel an injectable treatment is inappropriate. This conviction has grown over the many years it has taken to become a consultant dermatologist (I am not afraid to admit that I'm now a much better doctor – and communicator – than I was ten years ago). Unfortunately, there are many practitioners out there who lack the professional experience, and the confidence that naturally comes with that experience, to say no. And even worse are the greedy, and frankly unethical, types who coerce you into buying treatments for their own financial gain.

Personally, I think that where injectable treatments are concerned, you will be in safe hands with a properly accredited dermatologist or plastic surgeon who carries out these procedures. They have the specialist understanding their extensive training provides, but also the experience and confidence to be forthright about what you need. And as they usually have mixed practices – treating everything ranging from potentially fatal cancer to fine lines and wrinkles – they are better able to remain grounded in reality and maintain the 'aesthetic eye' essential in providing good results from injectable treatments.

In terms of my own speciality, I will outline how best to do this in chapter 9, 'Finding a Dermatologist'.

a) Other uses of dermal filler

Lip augmentation: Dermal filler can be used in patients looking for lip augmentation. Hyaluronic acid fillers are used most commonly, and when injected into the lips can enhance shape, structure or volume. The results typically last six months and need to be repeated for as long as one wants their effects. Lip fillers are not suitable for everyone and an assessment of facial shape needs to be made first otherwise there is a risk that the end result will look unnatural. This is a popular clinic procedure in younger patients, particularly those in their twenties. It does, however, have a role in older patients also. Ageing of the lip results in a downturn of the mouth. In profile, the lips recede with age, particularly the lower lip, and lip definition is lost. Filler can be used around the mouth to correct this.

Hand rejuvenation: It is often said that looking at someone's hands is a reliable giveaway of their real age. Volume loss in the hands as we get older gives them a sunken appearance, and bones, tendons and veins become more visible. Filler containing calcium hydroxylapatite is commonly used and injected into the backs of the hands. This is massaged and swelling can occur for a few days. The filler lasts about six months or so. This is a relatively safe area to inject, with few side effects.

SKIN RESURFACING TECHNIQUES

So Botox will deal with some lines and filler with sagging and volume loss. But what about the texture of the skin itself? As skin ages, it will also develop lots of fine lines, uneven skin tone, redness and pigmentation. Skin resurfacing techniques exist to deal with these changes.

Chemical peels

Chemical peels are a medical or clinic-grade procedure in which a chemical solution is applied to the skin to create accelerated exfoliation and peeling. The new skin is often smoother and less pigmented than the skin which comes away. Chemical peels can be used for treating signs of ageing, such as lines and pigmentation, in addition to skin disorders such as acne.

Chemical peels are usually divided into three main types: superficial, medium and deep. Superficial peels are the mildest and affect only the upper layer of the skin (epidermis). Medium-depth peels act on the upper and middle skin layers; deep peels penetrate deeper still.

The process begins with cleansing of the skin. The chemical solution is then applied to the face, or other area to be treated, usually for five to ten minutes. It is possible to feel a burning or stinging sensation during this time. With superficial peels, there is minor redness and the skin may feel tight for a few hours afterwards. Minor skin shedding occurs for a few days. Medium and deep peels have longer recovery times and can result in skin redness, swelling and peeling for seven to fourteen days.

Following a peel, the skin is more sensitive to sunshine and care must be taken to protect the skin by wearing high-factor SPF (minimum 30) for at least four weeks. Peels can be repeated at regular intervals and are extremely helpful in treating changes in skin tone and texture.

a) Superficial chemical peels

These are generally the safest and are usually used in all skin types including darker skin. Often, a course of peels is required to obtain the best clinical response. Common peeling agents include the alpha-hydroxy acids (AHAs) such as glycolic, lactic, mandelic, pyruvic and citric acid. These products can also have a role in anti-ageing skincare but percentages available in over-the-counter products that you use at home are usually significantly less than in clinic-grade peels, so the results will never be quite the same.

Other agents used for superficial peeling include the beta-hydroxy acid, salicylic acid. This is particularly good for acne but should be avoided in pregnancy. Tretinoin, trichloroacetic acid (10–25 per cent) and Jessner's solution (resorcinol 14 per cent, lactic acid 14 per cent and salicylic acid 14 per cent) are other commonly used agents for superficial peels.

b) Medium and deep chemical peels

These traditionally use trichloroacetic acid in high percentages or an agent known as phenol. Deeper peels can be used for a number of anti-ageing concerns but have a longer recovery time associated with them.

With all chemical peels, there is a risk of reactivation of cold sores, pigmentation changes and, rarely, scarring (often on the lower face). It is vitally important that the right peel for the right problem and the right skin type is chosen.

Light and laser treatments

Light and laser systems are extremely effective at skin rejuvenation, treating pigmentation, redness, lines and wrinkles – in essence, resurfacing the skin.

Whilst many establishments offer laser treatments, training can be variable and it is always better to seek treatment with an experienced doctor or laser dermatologist. The bonus of seeing a dermatologist is the expertise; he or she is fully trained in diagnosing and treating all skin conditions. For example, when having freckles treated, it is crucial that your treating practitioner has the training to recognize whether the skin lesion they are zapping away is genuinely a freckle rather than an early skin cancer known as lentigo maligna. I have seen first-hand, in clinic, the results of the mistakes that occur. Do your research on the reputability of both the clinic and the treating practitioner.

a) Light

Intense pulsed light (IPL) uses high-intensity pulses of light to target blood vessels and pigment in skin. It will improve the appearance of freckles, redness, age spots, facial lines and wrinkles. It is commonly used on the face, neck and décolleté.

The treatment lasts about twenty to thirty minutes and a course of four to six sessions at approximately monthly intervals is required. Protective eyewear should be worn by the practitioner and person being treated. The treatment is not painful but feels very much like hot rubber bands being flicked against the skin surface. After the treatment, the skin is red and can feel sensitive. There may be minor swelling or bruising and care must be taken in the sun for the following four weeks. This treatment is not suitable for darker skin types.

b) LED devices

LEDs and facials incorporating LED lights (usually red or blue light) have gained popularity in recent years. These are non-invasive and relatively safe treatments with minimal side effects. Data shows these can have some role in stimulating collagen production, improving skin texture and acting as an anti-inflammatory (e.g. in acne).

c) Lasers

Laser treatments remain one of the most effective ways of reversing the textural skin changes and pigmentation associated with ageing. Treatments have come a long way in the past few decades and technology is advancing rapidly in the number of options now available.

In the 1980s and 1990s, the use of a carbon dioxide laser for skin resurfacing was extremely popular. These would literally ablate or vaporize tissue allowing for new, healthy skin to grow through. They were associated with significant recovery time and marked swelling, redness and skin sloughing. This could take two to four weeks but produced the best cosmetic outcomes.

As technology changed, the use of 'non-ablative' lasers gained favour. Non-ablative lasers leave the upper layer of skin, the epidermis, intact but damage the lower dermis. They have very little recovery time but are less effective than the traditional 'ablative' lasers (e.g. KTP 532 laser, Nd:YAG 1320nm laser).

Fractional lasers then came along in the early 2000s and changed the way lasers were used in the skin-care arena. They work by targeting both the epidermis and dermis using a laser beam divided into many small, deep columns. These areas are known as microthermal treatment zones (MTZs). New collagen production occurs in the MTZs whilst the untreated areas in between speed up wound healing. This results in a faster recovery process than if all the tissue had been heated. Fractional lasers can be ablative or non-ablative. Standard recovery can take a few days.

Lasers are a complex area and care needs to be taken with their use, particularly in darker skin types as there is a risk of causing problems with pigmentation. They remain one of the most effective ways to treat facial lines and wrinkles, sun damage, pigmentation and acne scarring. Compared to the other methods discussed in this chapter, they can also be more expensive. A proper consultation with a laser dermatologist or specialist should take place before any treatments are carried out. Often, a laser test patch is required before treatment.

OTHER SKIN REJUVENATION TECHNIQUES

Radio-frequency devices

These are non-invasive devices that deliver radio-frequency energy to the skin; examples include Thermage, Pelleve and Accent. They generate heat in the deeper skin layers which causes collagen disruption and new collagen formation. This will result in skin tightening and is commonly used to treat the jowls, jawline, neck and wrinkles around the eye area. It can be useful for those aged thirty to fifty with skin sagging and can safely be used on any skin type. It will not affect textural or pigmentation changes of the skin as it is primarily a skin-tightening procedure. There can be some redness after the procedure which usually settles within an hour. Normal activities can be resumed almost straight away.

High-Intensity Focused Ultrasound (HIFU)

Skin tightening and lifting was first introduced to the market with a device called Ulthera. A hand-piece is used to deliver concentrated ultrasound energy to the deeper skin layers, stimulating collagen production. The treatment is beneficial for those aged thirty to fifty and in people who do not want surgical intervention. It is commonly used to treat sagging of the face and neck and to tighten the jawline. The procedure is uncomfortable, and often painkillers are administered beforehand. Results are effective and last for at least a year, but it can take three months or more from the point of treatment to see full benefit. There is some redness immediately after treatment which settles quickly, and normal activities can be resumed straight away. HIFU should be carried out by a medical practitioner.

Microneedling

Microneedling is a treatment offered by a spectrum of people including beauticians, aestheticians, nurses and doctors. It is a minimally invasive procedure which is sometimes known as collagen induction therapy. It is used most commonly for facial rejuvenation and mild acne scarring; it also has very limited use in stretch marks (striae). The skin is numbed with a topical cream for about thirty minutes prior to treatment. Following this, a device with fine needles is used to make multiple micro-injuries to the skin. This controlled injury triggers the body to produce new collagen. The procedure is well-tolerated but multiple sessions are often required. It is not as effective as laser treatments.

Platelet-rich Plasma (PRP) therapy

PRP therapy has gained much coverage through its well-publicized celebrity fan club. However, it existed in the medical arena for some time, particularly in orthopaedics and sports medicine, before it gained popularity for cosmetic uses.

Blood contains a number of cell types, of which platelets are one. Platelets are involved in blood clotting but also contain a number of growth factors and chemicals known as cytokines that can stimulate healing (e.g. epidermal growth factor, platelet-derived growth factor, transforming growth factor-beta). In PRP, your blood is taken and processed to make it rich in platelets. These are then activated and injected back into the skin with the intention of improving wrinkles and sun damage.

Scientific data surrounding PRP is still lacking, but it certainly seems to be showing promise for skin rejuvenation, wound healing and hair loss. It can also be combined with other treatments such as microneedling and laser.

Clearly, a full approach to anti-ageing requires knowledge and skill in being able to administer a number of techniques and combining different forms of treatment. I would always recommend choosing a doctor based on their wide scope of skills. It is all too easy to be sold a specific treatment as the best, simply because it is the only treatment a particular clinic may have to offer (e.g. microneedling for scars as there is no access to a laser). To get the best results, a thorough assessment of your needs is required to allow you to choose the best option for your time and budget.

This is exactly the thought process I go through when choosing a practitioner to do my anti-ageing treatments. I'm not ashamed to say that I've had Botox, fillers, Ulthera, chemical peels and lasers at different points in my life. Some have been to satisfy curiosity (e.g. Botox), whereas others were to deal with specific skin concerns (e.g. lasers for acne scarring). Over the years, I have had a number of these treatments and no doubt I'll have more as I grow older; this is a choice I have made and feel comfortable with. The added bonus is that I now know what it's like to experience these treatments, not just administer them!

8

MOLES AND SKIN CANCER

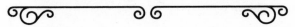

Dermatologists like to talk about skin cancer. A lot. It is one area of skin health that we do not want to ignore or miss. Rates of skin cancer in the UK have been rising significantly since the 1970s. Its incidence is thought to have increased as much as 360 per cent during this time.

Why is this? Well, since the 1970s we have seen an increase in the accessibility of foreign travel and budget holidays in the sun. The desire to be tanned has become popular and tanning bed usage more prevalent. Combine this with the thinning ozone layer in parts of the world and you can see how the problem has developed. Limiting ultraviolet light exposure remains the most important preventable factor in skin cancer. Something to think about.

There are three main types of skin cancer: melanoma, basal cell carcinoma and squamous cell carcinoma.

MELANOMA

This is the fifth most common cancer in the UK. It develops from the pigment-producing cells in the skin, known as melanocytes. Melanoma can develop as a new mole on the skin (the majority) or within a pre-existing mole.

What are the risk factors?

Ultraviolet light from the sun or from artificial tanning beds is the single biggest culprit. Other risk factors include fair skin, multiple sunburns, family history of melanoma in close relatives, conditions that cause a weakened immune system and the presence of lots of moles.

How dangerous is melanoma?

The reason we worry about melanoma is its ability to spread to other organs, or 'metastasize'. Melanoma has the potential to spread to the liver, lungs, bone and brain, where it can potentially be fatal. The good news is that most melanomas are picked up at an early stage, well before this happens.

How can I reduce my risk of melanoma?

There is no national screening programme in the UK for melanoma. Your best chance of picking up a melanoma early is to know the signs and when to seek medical attention. I can't stress enough how vital this is. For those who have private healthcare, many choose to have annual mole checks performed by a dermatologist as part of their preventative health screening.

Educating yourself and your loved ones is key in bringing down rates of melanoma. The skin is a visual organ and any surface changes should, in theory, be easier to pick up than disease in some other organ, which would require an internal scan.

What should I look out for when checking my own or others' skin?

The acronym ABCDE is used most commonly as a tool for evaluating moles. If a mole shows any of these features, it warrants review by a dermatologist.

- *Asymmetry*: One half of the mole is different from the other.

- *Border*: The mole's edge is irregular, scalloped or poorly defined.
- *Colour*: There is uneven colour or variable colours within the mole.
- *Diameter*: The mole is bigger than 6mm in size.
- *Evolving*: The mole is changing in its size, shape or colour.

Other signs to look out for include any new moles or a mole that looks significantly different from the others (known as the 'ugly duckling' sign). The most common site for developing a melanoma in a male is the back, and in a female, the legs.

The tricky thing is that not all changing moles are indicative of skin cancer, and actually most moles are harmless. It can be normal for moles to change in number and appearance; some can also disappear over time. Hormonal changes during puberty and pregnancy can cause moles to increase in number and become darker.

How should I check my skin for moles?

Most dermatologists recommend you should examine your skin yourself on a monthly basis. The ideal time is probably after a bath or shower in a well-lit room with the aid of a full-length mirror. Develop a system (e.g. from head to toe), first examining the front and then the back, to ensure that you do not miss a section of your body. It can be helpful to get a trusted person to look at your back and other hard-to-examine areas. Take care not to miss sites like the buttocks, genital area, palms and soles. Some people find taking photographs once a year a good way to have a record of their skin. The first few months will purely be an exercise in getting used to where your moles and blemishes are, and what is normal for your skin. This becomes easier over time, although it can be challenging for those with many moles.

What should I do if I'm worried about a mole?

If you have any concerns regarding a mole which is changing, it is important to seek medical attention. You should visit your GP who will either reassure you or refer you to a dermatologist, either on the NHS or privately if you have medical insurance. Alternatively, it is possible to see a private dermatologist directly. There are therefore multiple routes for seeking help depending on urgency and budget.

What will happen in my consultation with a dermatologist?

Your dermatologist will usually carry out a total body skin examination with the aid of a dermatoscope. This is essentially a magnifying light, which allows us to see the details of the mole much more clearly to make an assessment. If there is any concern, the worrying mole is removed under local anaesthetic and sent to the lab for analysis, which will check for cancer. The mole removal is a quick procedure that takes twenty to thirty minutes and usually involves stitches to close the wound.

If the lab results show that my mole was cancerous, what happens next?

The majority of people who have a melanoma removed will have no further problems. However, this does rely on the melanoma being removed at an early stage. The bottom line remains that the earlier the melanoma is caught, the better the survival rate.

I have seen mole clinics on the high street. Are these a good idea?

I'd advise caution when considering mole clinics. I often see patients that have previously been to such private clinics and learned that, frighteningly, many of these clinics do not have an in-house dermatologist and simply use a computerized machine to decide if a mole is worrying or not. If the machine flags the mole as a problem, they are then advised to see a dermatologist elsewhere.

From my point of view, there are a few issues with this, all of which I have seen first-hand:

- The technology is not sufficiently sophisticated at present to make a machine that is more reliable than a dermatologist.
- The machine is not able to look at your body as a whole and put what is seen into context. For example, my moles may all look slightly odd, but they are all the 'same odd'; therefore, that may simply be normal for me. The machine is unable to use that human context.
- There are many situations where you might be told you have an 'abnormal' mole by machine mapping and then find out there is no in-house dermatologist to look at it or remove it. This generates a great deal of anxiety whilst you then have to find another clinic with a dermatologist. It has happened on several occasions that a supposed 'abnormal' mole is harmless but the worry it has created results in its removal, an unnecessary procedure and scar. My advice

would be to always get your mole reviewed by a dermatologist if there is concern, and cut out these middle steps.

- Even worse, in some of these clinics a doctor without proper dermatological training will proceed to remove a mole purely because the machine flagged it, even though an inspection from a dermatologist would have indicated there was no need for concern, let alone surgery. Personal experience shows that this occurs surprisingly often.

NON-MELANOMA SKIN CANCER

There are two main types of non-melanoma skin cancer: basal cell and squamous cell carcinoma. Ultraviolet light, usually from the sun, is yet again the most common cause of their development. These types of cancer usually look like scaly patches or pink bumps on the skin that fail to heal. They can become scabby and bleed, and are occasionally tender to touch.

Non-melanoma skin cancers can develop on any part of the body but are usually seen on sun-exposed sites such as the face, neck, forearms and hands. In men, they can develop on the scalp, especially if there is little hair to provide protection. They are the result of chronic sun damage over the years and usually affect people in their fifties onwards. However, you can see them in younger individuals, particularly if there has been a lot of sun exposure. These types of cancer have a much lower likelihood of spread compared to melanoma, and treatment is usually curative, often with surgery.

If you notice a non-healing patch of skin that fails to settle after a few weeks, it is worthwhile seeing your GP for evaluation to exclude these types of cancer. If there is concern, you will be referred to a dermatologist.

PREVENTION

Sun protection is the single most effective method for reducing your risk of skin cancer. This is particularly important if you have risk factors such as fair skin, family history or many moles.

Cover up

This remains your first-line option in protecting against the sun. This should be something you think about on a hot, sunny day in the UK, whilst on a tropical holiday or even when participating in outdoor sport. Clothing, hats and sunglasses all have a role to play.

Shelter

Ideally try and stay out of the sun during peak daylight hours, when the sun is most likely to cause burning. This is usually between 11 a.m. and 3 p.m. Try and seek shade during these times.

Sunscreen

Look for a broad-spectrum sunscreen that offers protection against both UVA and UVB rays from the sun. This should be a minimum of SPF 15–30. Sunscreens can be of two kinds – mineral and chemical. Chemical sunscreens need to be applied at least twenty minutes before going outdoors; mineral sunscreens contain zinc and titanium, and work as soon as they are applied. Sunscreens need to be reapplied every ninety minutes to get the stated protection factor on the bottle and most of us are guilty of not reapplying it as frequently as we should. Also remember to reapply after swimming and sweating. It is best to avoid once-daily formulations, as they are not likely to be as effective.

Most of us also do not use the correct quantities of sunscreen for it to be effective. Sunscreen needs to be used on all areas not covered by clothing. About one shot-glass-full (or 35ml) should be about right for an average-sized adult. A rough rule of thumb is about a teaspoon per body area: one teaspoon for your face, head and neck, one for each arm, one for each leg, one for your chest and abdomen and one for your back and the back of the neck. Don't forget your ears and the tops of your feet; these are commonly missed sites.

Many people do not use sunscreen on cloudy days. This is, in fact, the time we often see the worst sunburn due to false security that there is no sunshine around. The truth is that you still need your sunscreen on cloudy days.

I often get asked if it is necessary to wear sunscreen every day, including the winter months. It is true that there is less UVB radiation in the winter in the UK, the main ray that can cause burning. However, as many skin cancers develop due to cumulative UV exposure, it is worthwhile getting into the habit of wearing sunscreen on your exposed sites daily. For those who are concerned, it will also have benefits for your skin from an anti-ageing perspective.

Special care needs to be taken with small children in the sun. Blistering sunburn in childhood can double a person's risk of developing melanoma in later life. Young skin is particularly vulnerable to the effects of ultraviolet radiation. Babies below the age of six months have little melanin in their skin and their skin is too sensitive for the use of sunscreens. It is therefore important that young babies are not left in direct sunlight. After six months of age, sunscreen is safe to apply.

SUNBURN

Despite one's best intentions, it is still possible to get caught out by the sun and get burnt. Sunburn causes direct damage to DNA, resulting in inflammation and death of skin cells. The skin can become hot, red, tender, swollen and blistered. This normally develops two to six hours after sun exposure and peaks at twelve to twenty-four hours. Clearly, this is not an ideal situation, but should it occur, it is important to know how to manage it.

1. Get out of the sun

This seems entirely obvious but is the single most important thing to do! Cover up all affected areas and stay out of the sun until sunburn heals. Wear loose cotton clothing that allows your skin to breathe.

2. Analgesia (pain control)

Take over-the-counter anti-inflammatory painkillers (e.g. ibuprofen). These not only reduce pain but also help with inflammation. They can be taken for forty-eight hours if there are no allergies.

3. Cool the skin

Take a bath rather than powerful shower, which can potentially damage the affected skin, particularly if there are blisters. Keep water temperature below lukewarm. Cold compresses against the skin (e.g. a towel dampened in cold water) may provide some relief.

4. Moisturize

After a bath or shower, use an unperfumed cream or lotion to soothe the skin. Repeated applications are necessary to reduce the appearance of peeling and this may need to be continued for several weeks. Aloe vera or soy-containing gels or lotions can be beneficial in soothing the skin. Aloe vera not only cools the skin but also acts as an anti-inflammatory. If possible, avoid using creams or lotions that contain petroleum, benzocaine or lidocaine. These can either trap heat in the skin or cause local skin irritation.

5. Drink water

Stay hydrated as sunburn can encourage fluid loss through the skin. Alcohol should ideally be avoided as it is a diuretic and can lead to further fluid loss and dehydration when you least need it.

6. Mild topical steroid

Using a relatively weak steroid such as 0.5 per cent or 1 per cent hydrocortisone purchased over the counter for forty-eight hours can reduce inflammation and itching associated with sunburn. This is best avoided in small children without medical advice.

7. Don't pick your blisters

Popping blisters can lead to infection and scarring – leave them alone! After a bath or shower, gently pat the skin dry, rather than vigorously rubbing with a towel, otherwise fragile blisters may break.

THE VITAMIN D SAGA

I have no doubt that many of you are reading my sun protection advice and thinking about how you are supposed to get your vitamin D if you follow these instructions.

The vitamin D story is incredibly complicated and has become messy and confused by the media and medical profession, resulting in much conflicting advice. Evidence shows that rigorous sun protection can lead to vitamin D deficiency but people like me still advise that dangers of sun exposure outweigh the benefits.

Vitamin D is a fat-soluble vitamin essential for maintaining bone health. It also provides protection against some types of cancer, heart disease, multiple sclerosis and diabetes, as well as having positive benefits for mood and well-being.

Unprotected sun exposure is the major source of vitamin D production for most of us. Sunlight, in particular UVB radiation, is needed for vitamin D synthesis in the skin. The amount of available UVB varies significantly depending on the time of day, season and latitude. Vitamin D production also varies from person to person, with pigmented skin types requiring a longer period of exposure to make the same quantity of vitamin D.

Most dermatologists agree that the time taken to make vitamin D in the skin is relatively short, and less than the time needed for skin to become red and burn. Of more interest and a less-commonly known fact is that continued sun exposure does NOT result in ongoing vitamin D production. After prolonged UVB exposure, vitamin D is converted into inactive substances. There is, therefore, little point sunbathing for long periods of time in order to 'top up' your level.

Current UK dermatology guidance recommends going outdoors for a few minutes around midday without sunscreen to improve vitamin D levels. Individuals are encouraged to recognize their own skin to get some idea of how long one can spend outdoors without burning. This time is clearly going to be shorter for someone with pale skin than a comparable person with dark skin.

One of the problems that we have in the UK is that due to our latitude we do not get sufficient UVB radiation to produce vitamin D from sunlight between October and March. So, firstly, it is worthwhile trying to improve vitamin D intake from dietary sources, particularly during the winter. Foods rich in vitamin D include oily fish (e.g. mackerel, salmon, sardines), fortified margarine and cereals, and egg yolks. Failing that, consider taking an oral supplement during this time of year. Total daily dose of vitamin D should be 800 IU.

Based on current data, the conclusion remains that there are safer ways to get enough vitamin D, which do not involve prolonged sun exposure. There is probably no benefit in over-supplementing or taking more than necessary, as high levels of vitamin D have also been linked to health issues.

9

FINDING A DERMATOLOGIST

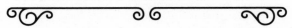

Now this may come as a shock – it does to me – but there is little regulation in the UK around the terms 'dermatologist', 'skin doctor' and 'skin specialist'. On a daily basis, I come across people calling themselves dermatologists or skin experts without appropriate training. The amount of times I see an expert quote in a glossy magazine or broadsheet by someone who has been labelled as a dermatologist without the qualification to back it up is staggering. Marketing and hype, unfortunately, is not limited to beauty products but extends to your doctor too.

Dermatologists in the UK spend several years as a junior doctor doing exams after they qualify from medical school. During this time, they gain experience in other disciplines – I did a variety of jobs as a young doctor in Cardiff, including cardiology, renal medicine, stroke and acute medicine. After this, applications are made for specialist training. Dermatology is a hugely competitive speciality to get into and many are left disappointed. After several years of following a strict dermatology curriculum and yet more exams, one completes specialist training and becomes a consultant dermatologist. Let's make no bones about it: the slog to the end is long and arduous.

What continues to amaze me is the audacity of those who have not done this training to use the label of 'dermatologist'. I would never say that I was a heart expert despite having done eight months as a junior doctor in cardiology. Dare I say it, but it is deceptive and fraudulent. It is there to deliberately mislead you into believing you are seeing a genuine expert. This is a controversial topic and one that ruffles feathers, particularly in the rather corrupt aesthetics industry – I have been accused of elitism in the past when pointing it out. But I beg to differ; it is about honesty and transparency. The general public has a right to know who is treating them and a right to know their level of expertise.

And why does it matter? Let me explain by example. A few months ago, I had a patient in her twenties come to see me. She had been to a beauty clinic to have a mole that she didn't like removed. The practitioner, lacking the wherewithal and training to recognize the danger signs, duly obliged and tried to burn the mole away with a laser. Unfortunately, the lesion continued to bleed and she attended my clinic for review some months later. It was a melanoma, the most dangerous type of skin cancer. In my books, this kind of situation should never arise.

Acne provides other good examples of skin mismanagement. There are many ways to treat it effectively: creams, tablets, isotretinoin, light and laser devices. Any dermatologist knows that once you see scarring, certain treatments are better than others. Yet I have lost count of how many patients come to see me having spent thousands elsewhere on skincare, chemical peels and light devices that simply do not provide long-term control. They have been frightened off using oral medications because of alleged side effects. And conveniently, of course, it is often the people scaremongering who have the least experience (if they even have any at all) in prescribing these medicines – medicines that can be used in a safe manner when under expert guidance.

Doing a weekend course does not make one a specialist. One needs to understand the skin in health and disease. It needs to be looked at in context with the rest of the human body and how it interacts with other organs. My job is not to sell treatments. A real dermatologist's skill comes from a deep understanding of skin and the ability to have a meaningful discussion regarding all treatment options, not just the new laser device that has received good PR in last night's tabloid.

So how do you check the credentials of your doctor? If you are in the UK and seeing a dermatologist on the NHS, this should be easy: if they have the title 'consultant derma-tologist', they are fully trained. In the US, make sure your dermatologist has board-certification (which is the equiva-lent of reaching consultant level). Other parts of the world will have similar accreditations and listings. If there is any uncertainty, ask for an official title; don't assume.

It is much harder in the private sector or if you choose to see a dermatologist for cosmetic reasons. Always start with doing your own research. Don't make any assump-tions about qualifications despite what you read in your favourite magazine or newspaper. You need to know with whom you are dealing, seeing through the guff of fancy websites and clever marketing strategies.

GUIDE TO CHOOSING A DERMATOLOGIST

General Medical Council (GMC) membership

If you are in the UK, check the GMC website: www.gmc-uk.org.

Every practising doctor with a licence to practise in the UK will be on this register. You just need the doctor's name to check them out. A qualified dermatologist will be listed here as 'on the specialist register for dermatology'; a qualified GP will be listed here as 'on the GP register'. If your treating skin expert is not on the specialist register, you need to ask why. It could simply be that a doctor has trained abroad with an equivalent qualification OR it could be a sign that they do not have the necessary training. If you don't ask, you won't find out. This is the single most important thing you must do.

Word of mouth

The next step is to speak to friends, neighbours, family and your GP. They can provide a wealth of knowledge and are likely to be able to guide you if they have had their own experiences with a dermatologist. There is huge strength in personal recommendation.

Check reviews

In the digital era, nearly all doctors will have some sort of Google footprint. There are a number of independent review sites available that provide feedback both from patients and from other medical colleagues. Think of it as a bit like TripAdvisor. If a doctor has a large number of reviews and the vast majority of these are positive, they are worthy of consideration.

Assess their website and other social media channels

You want to ensure the dermatologist you see is a good fit for your personality. It is much more common these days for doctors to have their own websites and easily accessible social media channels. If these are publicly available, have a quick look through and satisfy yourself that this is the doctor you want to go and see.

Dermatology is rapidly changing from how I recall it to have been when I was growing up. I took many trips to see various dermatologists as a child, and then in my teens and twenties, for both eczema and acne. My experience was very much of patriarchal figures who were able to deal with me medically but had little interest in my skincare, lifestyle or how rotten I felt. There is no doubt that my experience has been mirrored by many others, including a great many of my own patients.

A lack of interest in these other human factors and poor regulation in the aesthetics industry has resulted in mushrooming of 'pseudo-specialists' willing to address them but not necessarily with the same scientific understanding as a dermatologist. Luckily, times are now bringing in a new breed: incredibly competent, high-calibre dermatologists who also have the ability to unashamedly discuss your beauty, skincare and lifestyle needs. Do your research and make sure you end up with the very best your skin deserves. Do it, in the words of a rather famous French cosmetics company, 'Because you're worth it.'

SOME FINAL THOUGHTS

Working with skin has privileged me with the unique position of being a qualified dermatologist with a healthy and unbiased interest in beauty, cosmetics and aesthetics. To be able to analyse scientific data in the skincare industry is of huge benefit in critically evaluating the products. Don't forget, after all, that the market is there to sell; it is not there for your interest.

Consumers need genuine guidance on what will really help their specific skincare needs. One size does not fit all and expert advice is vital to manoeuvre through celebrity endorsements and poorly hidden advertorials in magazines or newspapers. On a personal note, it drives me mad seeing the amount of bad information out there, and madder still when it's coming from someone pretending to be an expert.

If there's anything you take away from this book, I hope it's this: check your doctor's credentials and start to become clued up on common skincare ingredients. Skincare does not have to be complicated or expensive. Hopefully, much of what you have read herein demonstrates this and arms you with the knowledge to go forward and obtain what your skin really needs in order to shine.

ACKNOWLEDGEMENTS

The biggest thank you goes to my rock – my husband, Nik Kyriakides, for his never-ending love and unwavering support of everything I do. This book would not have been possible without him.

I would also like to make a special mention to my sister, Arti, for her positivity in all my endeavours, and my friend and mentor, Nisith Sheth, for all his encouragement and guidance over the years.

Lastly, thank you to my editors and everyone at Penguin who has helped shape this book and bring it to life.